Second
Edition

Nurse Executive

Review and Resource Manual

CONTINUING EDUCATION SOURCE

NURSING CERTIFICATION REVIEW MANUAL

CLINICAL PRACTICE RESOURCE

Al Rundio, PhD, DNP, RN, APRN, ANP, ACNP, ACNS, CARN-AP, NEA-BC, DPNAP

Virginia Wilson, PhD(c), MSN, RN, NEA-BC, NE-BC

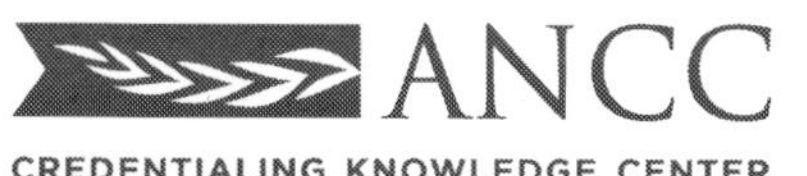

Conferences.
Consultation.
Education.

Library of Congress Cataloging-in-Publication Data

Nurse Executive review and resource manual. - 2nd ed. / by Al Rundio and Virginia Wilson.
p. ; cm.
Rev. ed. of: Nurse Executive review and resource manual / by Al Rundio and Virginia Wilson... [et al.]. 1st ed. 2010.
Includes bibliographical references and index.
ISBN 9781935213383 (alk. paper)
I. Al Rundio. Virginia Wilson. American Nurses Credentialing Center. II. Nursing Executive review and resource manual. II. Title.
[DNLM: 1. Nurse Executive–methods–United States–Examination Questions. 2. Nurse Executive–methods–United States–Handbooks. 3. Nurse Executive–methods–United States–Outlines. WY 18.2]

618.92'00231–dc23

2012047149

The American Nurses Credentialing Center (ANCC), a subsidiary of the American Nurses Association (ANA), provides individuals and organizations throughout the nursing profession with the resources they need to achieve practice excellence. ANCC's internationally renowned credentialing programs certify nurses in specialty practice areas; recognize healthcare organizations for promoting safe, positive work environments through the Magnet Recognition Program® and the Pathway to Excellence ® Program; and accredit providers of continuing nursing education. In addition, ANCC's Institute for Credentialing Innovation provides leading-edge information and education services and products to support its core credentialing programs.

ISBN 13: 9781935213659

8515 Georgia Ave., Suite 400
Silver Spring, MD 20910

NURSE EXECUTIVE REVIEW AND RESOURCE MANUAL, 2ND EDITION

JUNE 2013

The healthcare services delivery system is a volatile marketplace demanding superior knowledge, clinical skills, and competencies from all registered nurses. Nursing autonomy of practice and nurse career marketability and mobility in the new century hinge on affirming the profession's formative philosophy, which places a priority on a lifelong commitment to the principles of education and professional development. The knowledge base of nursing theory and practice is expanding, and while care has been taken to ensure the accuracy and timeliness of the information presented in the **Nurse Executive Review and Resource Manual**, clinicians are advised to always verify the most current national guidelines and recommendations and to practice in accordance with professional standards of care used with regard to the unique circumstances that apply in each practice situation. In addition, the editors wish to note that provision of information in this text does not imply an endorsement of any particular products, procedures or services.

Therefore, the authors, editors, American Nurses Association (ANA), American Nurses Association's Publishing (ANP), American Nurses Credentialing Center (ANCC), and the Credentialing Knowledge Center cannot accept responsibility for errors or omissions, or for any consequences or liability, injury, and/or damages to persons or property from application of the information in this manual and make no warranty, express or implied, with respect to the contents of the **Nurse Executive Review and Resource Manual**. Completion of this manual does not guarantee that the reader will pass the certification exam. The practice examination questions are not a requirement to take a certification examination. The practice examination questions cannot be used as an indicator of results on the actual certification.

Published by: American Nurses Credentialing Center
Credentialing Knowledge Center
8515 Georgia Avenue, Suite 400
Silver Spring, MD 20910-3402
www.nursecredentialing.org

INTRODUCTION TO THE CONTINUING EDUCATION (CE) CONTACT HOUR APPLICATION PROCESS FOR *NURSE EXECUTIVE REVIEW AND RESOURCE MANUAL, 2ND EDITION*

The Credentialing Knowledge Center now offers the continuing education contact hours for this manual online at www.NursingWorld.org, the American Nurses Association's website. This process involves answering approximately 25–30 questions that test knowledge of the information contained within this manual. The continuing education contact hours can be completed at any time and a certificate can be printed from the website immediately upon successful completion of the test.

After studying the manual and given an online multiple-choice test, the exam candidate will be able to:

1. Pass the posttest with at least 75% of the answers correct.
2. Select responses to test questions based on key principles, standards of practice, and theoretical basis of nursing practice.
3. Choose accepted therapeutic interventions in answering questions related to quality nursing practice.
4. Utilize direct and indirect professional role responsibilities and applications regarding nursing practice in answering test questions.

Upon completion of this manual *and* the online CE test, a nurse can receive a total of 16 continuing education contact hours at a price of $32, only $2 per CE. (ANA members receive a discount on CEs.) **The entire process—online test and evaluation form**—must be completed by June 30, 2016 **in order to receive credit.** To begin the process, please e-mail **revmanuals@ana.org**. Your patience with this process is greatly appreciated.

Inquiries or Comments

If you have any questions about the CE contact hours, please email the Credentialing Knowledge Center at revmanuals@ana.org. You may also mail any comments to Editorial Project Manager, at the address listed below.

Duplicate CE Certificates

Once you have successfully passed the CE test, you may go back and re-print your certificate as often as you wish.

Conflicts of Interest

A conflict of interest occurs when an individual has an opportunity to affect educational content about healthcare products or services of a commercial company with which she/he has a financial relationship.

The planners and presenters of this CNE activity have disclosed no relevant financial relationships with any commercial companies pertaining to this activity.

Credentialing Knowledge Center
American Nurses Credentialing Center
Attn: Editorial Project Manager
8515 Georgia Avenue, Suite 400
Silver Spring, MD 20910-3492
Fax: (301) 628-5342

A maximum of 16 contact hours may be earned by learners who successfully complete this continuing nursing education activity.

ANA's Center for Continuing Education and Professional Development is accredited as a provider of continuing nursing education by the American Nurses Credentialing Center's Commission on Accreditation.

ANCC Provider Number 0023.

ANA's Center for Continuing Education and Professional Development is approved by the California Board of Registered Nursing, Provider Number CEP6178 for 19.2 contact hours (50 minute contact hour).

The ANA Center for Continuing Education and Professional Development includes ANCC's Credentialing Knowledge Center.

CONTENTS

CHAPTER 1

TAKING THE CERTIFICATION EXAMINATION

When you sign up to take a national certification exam, you will be instructed to go online and review the testing and renewal handbook (www.nursecredentialing.org/documents/certification/application/generaltestingandrenewalhandbook.aspx). Review it carefully and be sure to bookmark the site so you can refer to it frequently. It contains information on test content and sample questions. This is critical information; it will give you insight into the nature of the test. The agency will send you information about the test site; keep this in a safe place until needed.

GENERAL SUGGESTIONS FOR PREPARING FOR THE EXAM

Step One: Control Your Anxiety

Everyone experiences anxiety when faced with taking the certification exam.

- Remember, your program was designed to prepare you to take this exam.
- Your instructors took a similar exam, and have probably talked to students who took exams more recently, so they know how to help you prepare.
- Taking a review course or setting up your own study plan will help you feel more confident about taking the exam.

Step Two: Do Not Listen to Gossip About the Exam

A large volume of information exists about the tests based on reports from people who have taken the exams in the past. Because information from the testing facilities is limited, it is hard to ignore this gossip.

- Remember that gossip about the exam that you hear from others is not verifiable.
- Because this gossip is based on the imperfect memory of people in a stressful situation, it may not be very accurate.
- People tend to remember those items testing content with which they are less comfortable; for instance, those with a limited background in women's health may say that the exam was "all women's health." In fact, the exam blueprint ensures that the exam covers multiple content areas without overemphasizing any one.

Step Three: Set Reasonable Expectations for Yourself

- Do not expect to know everything.
- Do not try to know everything in great detail.
- You do not need a perfect score to pass the exam.
- Learn the general rules, not the exceptions.

Step Four: Prepare Mentally and Physically

- While you are getting ready to take the exam, take good physical care of yourself.
- Get plenty of sleep and exercise, and eat well while preparing for the exam.
- These things are especially important while you are studying and immediately before you take the exam.

Step Five: Access Current Knowledge

General Content

You will be given a list of general topics that will be on the exam when you register to take it. In addition, examine the table of contents of this book and the test content outline, available at www.nursecredentialing.org/cert/TCOs.html.

- What content do you need to know?
- How well do you know these subjects?

Take a Review Course

- Taking a review course is an excellent way to assess your knowledge of the content that will be included in the exam.
- If you plan to take a review course, take it well before the exam so you will have plenty of time to master any areas of weakness the course uncovers.
- If you are prepared for the exam, you will not hear anything new in the course. You will be familiar with everything that is taught.
- If some topics in the review course are new to you, concentrate on these in your studies.
- People have a tendency to study what they know; it is rewarding to study something and feel a mastery of it! Unfortunately, this will not help you master unfamiliar content. Be sure to use a review course to identify your areas of strength and weakness, then concentrate on the weaknesses.

Depth of Knowledge

- How much do you need to know about a subject?
- You cannot know everything about a topic.
- Study the information sent to you from the testing agency, what you were taught in school, what is covered in this text, and the general guidelines given in this chapter.
- Look at practice tests designed for the exam. Practice tests for other exams will not be helpful.

Step Six: Institute a Systematic Study Plan

Develop Your Study Plan

- Write up a formal plan of study.
  - Include topics for study, timetable, resources, and methods of study that work for you.
  - Decide whether you want to organize a study group or work alone.
  - Schedule regular times to study.
  - Avoid cramming; it is counterproductive. Try to schedule your study periods in 1-hour increments.
- Identify resources to use for studying. To prepare for the examination, you should have the following materials on your shelf:
  - This review book.
  - Your class notes.
  - Other important sources, including information from the testing facility, favorite journal articles, notes from a review course, and practice tests.
  - Consult the bibliography on the test blueprint. When studying less familiar material, it is helpful to study using the same references that the testing center uses.
- You will need to know facts and be able to interpret and analyze this information utilizing critical thinking.

Personalize Your Study Plan

- How do you learn best?
  - If you learn best by listening or talking, attend a review course or discuss topics with a colleague.
- Read everything the test facility sends you as soon as you receive it and several times during your preparation period. It will give you valuable information to help guide your study.
- Identify a specific place with good lighting and set it aside for studying. Find a quiet place with no distractions. Assemble your study materials.

Implement Your Study Plan

You must have basic content knowledge. In addition, you must be able to use this information to think critically and make decisions based on facts.

- Refer to your study plan regularly.
- Stick to your schedule.
- Take breaks when you get tired.
- If you start procrastinating, get help from a friend or reorganize your study plan.
- It is not necessary to follow your plan rigidly. Adjust as you learn what areas need more focus and time.
- Memorize the basics of the content areas you will be required to know.

Focus on General Material

- Most of what you need to know is basic material that does not require constant updating.
- You do not need to worry about the latest information being published as you are studying for the exam. Remember, it can take 6 to 12 months for new information to be incorporated into test questions.

Pace Your Studying

- Stop studying for the examination when you are starting to feel overwhelmed and look at what is bothering you. Then make changes.
- Break overwhelming tasks into smaller tasks that you know you can do.
- Stop and take breaks while studying.

Work With Others

- Talk with classmates about your preparation for the exam.
- Keep in touch with classmates, and help each other stick to your study plans.
- If your classmates become anxious, do not let their anxiety affect you. Walk away if you need to.
- Do not believe bad stories you hear about other people's experiences with previous exams.
- Remember, you know as much as anyone about what will be on the next exam!

Consider a Study Group

- Study groups can provide practice in analyzing cases, interpreting questions, and critical thinking.
    - You can discuss a topic and take turns presenting cases for the group to analyze.
    - Study groups also can provide moral support and help you continue studying.

Step Seven: Strategies Immediately Before the Exam

Final Preparation Suggestions

- Use practice exams when studying to get accustomed to the exam format and time restrictions.
  - Many books that are labeled as review books are simply a collection of examination questions.
  - If you have test anxiety, such practice tests may help alleviate the anxiety.
  - Practice tests can help you learn to judge the time it should take you to complete the exam.
  - Practice tests are useful for gaining experience in analyzing questions.
  - Books of questions may not uncover the gaps in your knowledge that a more systematic content review text will reveal.
  - If you feel that you don't know enough about a topic, refer to a text to learn more. After you feel that you have learned the topic, practice questions are a wonderful tool to help improve your test-taking skills.
- Know your test-taking style.
  - Do you rush through the exam without reading the questions thoroughly?
  - Do you get stuck and dwell on a question for a long time?
  - You should spend about 45 to 60 seconds per question and finish with time to review the questions you were not sure about.
  - Be sure to read the question completely, including all four answer choices. Choice "a" may be good, but "d" may be best.

The Night Before the Exam

- Be prepared to get to the exam on time.
  - Know the test site location and how long it takes to get there.
  - Take a "dry run" beforehand to make sure you know how to get to the testing site, if necessary.
  - Get a good night's sleep.
  - Eat sensibly.
  - Avoid alcohol the night before.
  - Assemble the required material—two forms of identification, pencil, and watch. Both IDs must match the name on the application, and one photo ID is preferred.
  - Know the exam room rules.
    - You will be given scratch paper, which will be collected at the end of the exam.
    - Nothing else is allowed in the exam room.

- You will be required to put papers, backpacks, etc., in a corner of the room or in a locker.
- No water or food will be allowed.
- You will be allowed to walk to a water fountain and go to the bathroom one at a time.

The Day of the Exam

- Get there early. You must arrive to the test center at least 15 minutes before your scheduled appointment time. If you are late, you may not be admitted.
- Think positively. You have studied hard and are well-prepared.
- Remember your anxiety reduction strategies.

Specific Tips for Dealing With Anxiety

Test anxiety is a specific type of anxiety. Symptoms include upset stomach, sweaty palms, tachycardia, trouble concentrating, and a feeling of dread. But there are ways to cope with test anxiety.

- There is no substitute for being well-prepared.
- Practice relaxation techniques.
- Avoid alcohol, excess coffee, caffeine, and any new medications that might sedate you, dull your senses, or make you feel agitated.
- Take a few deep breaths and concentrate on the task at hand.

Focus on Specific Test-Taking Skills

To do well on the exam, you need good test-taking skills in addition to knowledge of the content and ability to use critical thinking.

All Certification Exams Are Multiple Choice

- Multiple-choice tests have specific rules for test construction.
- A multiple-choice question consists of three parts: the information (or stem), the question, and the four possible answers (one correct and three distracters).
- Careful analysis of each part is necessary. Read the entire question before answering.
- Practice your test-taking skills by analyzing the practice questions in this book and on the ANCC website.

Analyze the Information Given

- Do not assume you have more information than is given.
- Do not overanalyze.

- Remember, the writer of the question assumes this is all of the information needed to answer the question.
- If information is not given, it is not relevant and will not affect the answer.
- Do not make the question more complicated than it is.

What Kind of Question Is Asked?

- Are you supposed to recall a fact, apply facts to a situation, or understand and differentiate between options?
  - Read the question while thinking about what the writer is asking.
  - Look for key words or phrases that lead you (see Figure 1–1). These help determine what kind of answer the question requires.

FIGURE 1–1.
EXAMPLES OF KEY WORDS AND PHRASES

▸ avoid	▸ initial	▸ most
▸ best	▸ first	▸ significant
▸ except	▸ contributing to	▸ likely
▸ not	▸ appropriate	▸ of the following
		▸ most consistent with

Read All of the Answers

- If you are absolutely certain that answer "a" is correct as you read it, mark it, but read the rest of the question so you do not trick yourself into missing a better answer.
- If you are absolutely sure answer "a" is wrong, cross it off or make a note on your scratch paper and continue reading the question.
- After reading the entire question, go back, analyze the question, and select the best answer.
- Do not jump ahead.
- If the question asks you for an assessment, the best answer will be an assessment. Do not be distracted by an intervention that sounds appropriate.
- If the question asks you for an intervention, do not answer with an assessment.
- When two answer choices sound very good, the best one is usually the least expensive, least invasive way to achieve the goal. For example, if your answer choices include a physical exam maneuver or imaging, the physical exam maneuver is probably the better choice provided it will give the information needed.
- If the answers include two options that are the opposite of each other, one of the two is probably the correct answer.
- When numeric answers cover a wide range, a number in the middle is more likely to be correct.

- Watch out for distracters that are correct but do not answer the question, combine true and false information, or contain a word or phrase that is similar to the correct answer.
- Err on the side of caution.

Only One Answer Can Be Correct

- When more than one suggested answer is correct, you must identify the one that best answers the question asked.
- If you cannot choose between two answers, you have a 50% chance of getting it right if you guess.

Avoid Changing Answers

- Change an answer only if you have a compelling reason, such as you remembered something additional, or you understand the question better after rereading it.
- People change to a wrong answer more often than to a right answer.

Time Yourself to Complete the Whole Exam

- Do not spend a large amount of time on one question.
- If you cannot answer a question quickly, mark it and continue the exam.
- If time is left at the end, return to the difficult questions.
- Make educated guesses by eliminating the obviously wrong answers and choosing a likely answer even if you are not certain.
- Trust your instinct.
- Answer every question. There is no penalty for a wrong answer.
- Occasionally a question will remind you of something that helps you with a question earlier in the test. Look back at that question to see if what you are remembering affects how you would answer that question.

ABOUT THE CERTIFICATION EXAMS

The American Nurses Credentialing Center Computerized Exam

The ANCC examination is given only as a computer exam, and each exam is different.

The order of the questions is scrambled for every test, so even if two people are taking the same exam, the questions will be in a different order. The exam consists of 175 multiple-choice questions.

- 150 of the 175 questions are part of the test and how you answer will count toward your score; 25 are included to refine questions and will not be scored. You will not know which ones count, so treat all questions the same.
- You will need to know how to use a mouse, scroll by either clicking arrows on the scroll bar or using the up and down arrow keys, and perform other basic computer tasks.
- The exam does not require computer expertise.
- However, if you are not comfortable using a computer, you should practice using a mouse and computer beforehand so you do not waste time on the mechanics of using the computer.

Know What to Expect During the Test

- Each ANCC test question is independent of the other questions.
- For each case study, there is only one question. This means that a correct answer on any question does not depend on the correct answer to any other question.
- Each question has four possible answers. There are no questions asking for combinations of correct answers (such as "a and c") or multiple-multiples.
- You can skip a question and go back to it at the end of the exam.
- You cannot mark key words in the question or right or wrong answers. If you want to do this, use the scratch paper.
- You will get your results immediately, and a grade report will be provided upon leaving the testing site.

Internet Resources:

- ANCC website: www.nursecredentialing.org
- ANA Bookstore: www.nursesbooks.org. Catalog of ANA nursing scope and standards publications and other titles that may be listed on your test content outline
- National Guideline Clearinghouse: www.ngc.gov

CHAPTER 2

LEADERSHIP AND MANAGEMENT

LEADERSHIP THEORIES

The four leadership theories outlined here—trait, behavioral, contingency, and contemporary—have evolved over time and overlap to some extent.

Trait Theory

Leaders are assumed to possess certain traits that, if put into practice, result in success. *Trait theory* focuses on the characteristics of the leader. The initial set of leadership traits include drive, persistence, creative problem-solving, initiative, self-confidence, acceptance of the consequences of one's actions, resilience, tolerance, ability to influence others, and ability to structure social interactions. The list was further expanded to include such traits as intelligence, integrity, nonconformity, cooperativeness, and tact.

Behavioral Theory

In contrast to the characteristics that leaders possess, what leaders do, or how they behave, is the focus of behavioral theorists (see also "Organizational Theory" on page 15, specifically the work of Abraham Maslow, Frederick Herzberg, and their contemporaries).

The behaviorists categorize leaders by their style of practice:

- *Autocratic leaders* purport to change the behavior of subordinates through external control with the use of coercion, authority, punishment, and power.
- *Democratic leaders* appeal to the drive of their subordinates and influence change through participation, involvement of subordinates in goal-setting, and collaboration.
- *Permissive or laissez-faire leaders* use a "hands-off" approach and assume that people are able to make their own decisions and complete their work unaided by direction or facilitation.
- *Bureaucratic leaders* rely on organizational policies and rules to influence the behavior of their subordinates.

Autocratic and bureaucratic leaders assume that external motivators cause subordinates to change their behavior. Democratic and laissez-faire leaders believe that behavior change is internally inspired (i.e., internal locus of control).

To demonstrate the effectiveness of various styles of leadership, organizational psychologist Rensis Likert (Bateman & Snell, 2002) devised a four-quadrant model, known as System 4 Management, to illustrate the relationship between leadership behavior and outcomes. He describes leadership style according to the degree of involvement in decision-making managers invite from their subordinates. The terms Likert uses are similar to those noted above: autocratic, benevolent, consultative, and participative (democratic). His work shows that greater employee involvement translates to greater commitment to the organization and its objectives.

The managerial grid developed by Bateman and Snell (2002) is similar to Likert's quadrants and focuses on the varying degrees of concern managers have for production, people, or both. For example, impoverished leaders have a low concern for both people and production, while the team leaders show high concern in both of these dimensions.

Contingency Theory

While leaders may have an affinity for a particular style, no one style works effectively in every situation. For example, leaders who use a democratic style under conditions of stability may switch to an autocratic style in the face of an emergency that demands they take charge of a situation to achieve the best outcome. This ability to adapt one's approach to the situation at hand is labeled *contingency theory*, or situational leadership.

Organizational psychologist Fred Fiedler (as cited in Schermerhorn, Hunt, & Osborn, 2002) describes three leadership factors that influence outcomes:

1. ***Manager–follower relationships:*** To what degree does a manager enjoy the loyalty and support of her or his subordinates?
2. ***Task structure:*** To what degree is the task clearly described or are the operating procedures in place to guarantee a successful outcome?
3. ***Position power:*** To what degree is the manager able to administer rewards and punishment?

As an example, if a change in staffing practice is under consideration, it will have a better chance of acceptance if the leader–follower relationship is good, the task is structured, and the leader has high position power.

Paul Hersey and Ken Blanchard (as cited in Schermerhorn et al., 2002) took Fiedler's model a step further and added followers' willingness and readiness. They recommend that leaders consider the job and psychological maturity of their employees before deciding whether the leaders' task performance or maintenance (relationship) behaviors are more important. *Job maturity* refers to an employee's skill and technical knowledge relative to the job; *psychological maturity* refers to an employee's self-confidence and self-respect. Hersey and Blanchard posit that leaders in the situational leadership model use the following modes to move the agenda:

- *Leadership Style S1—High Task/Low Relationship (Telling):* The leader tells the worker what to do and provides close supervision.
- *Leadership Style S2—High Task/High Relationship (Selling):* The leader makes decisions and coaches followers; the leader provides opportunity for clarification.
- *Leadership Style S3—Low Task/High Relationship (Participating):* Both leader and follower participate in projects and decisions.
- *Leadership Style S4—Low Task/Low Relationship (Delegating):* The leader gives subordinates the freedom to make decisions and carry out plans.

In addition, subordinate readiness occurs along a continuum from low to high relative to ability and willingness. For example, the employee may be categorized as

- R1: Unable and unwilling; insecure;
- R2: Unable but willing; confident;
- R3: Able but unwilling; insecure; or
- R4: Able and willing; confident.

Vroom and Yetton's (as cited in Schermerhorn et al., 2002) expectancy model offers a prescriptive approach for managers to use when determining the amount of participation they should solicit from employees. The manager will adjust her or his leadership style in a given situation once answers to three key questions are clear:

1. Is all the information available to make the decision?
2. Is staff acceptance of the decision necessary to effective implementation?
3. Would the group's decision be one the leader could live with?

According to this model, the manager will then choose one of five decision-making approaches: tell, sell, consult, join, or delegate.

Contemporary Theories

Newer concepts of leadership are an amalgam of prior work in the field and include such descriptors as charismatic, transactional, transformational, connective, shared, and servant leadership. The complexity of today's work environment demands leader flexibility and adaptability as never before. There is no one "right" style of leadership.

Charismatic leaders are those who have the ability to engage others because of the power of their personalities. They inspire affection and emotional connection and may use the power of their personalities to advance revolutionary ideas.

Transactional leadership is derived from the principles of social-exchange theory. Social exchange implies that social, political, and psychological benefits exist in any relationship, including that of leader and follower, and that these benefits are reciprocal. Both manager and employee derive equal benefit from their relationship, and the interactions between them are meant to achieve and maintain balance (i.e., the status quo).

Transformational leadership is based on the principle that leaders transform the organization through contextual and cultural changes. The leader is aware of all that is going on in the organization. The transformational leader encourages risk-taking by subordinates and encourages an atmosphere of supportive trust and self-actualization for all employees. By contrast, transformational leadership moves people well beyond current reality. It seeks to gain support for change that is characterized as revolutionary. The leader is able to inspire others, to instill in them the belief that they can accomplish extraordinary things, often for the good of society. The American Nurses Credentialing Center's (ANCC) Magnet Recognition Program® is based on transformational leadership.

Connective leadership draws on the leader's ability to bring others together as a means of effecting change. Leaders in this category realize that the whole is greater than the sum of its parts and achieve results through collaboration, cooperation, coordination, and collegiality. They are able to foster interconnectedness among seemingly disparate groups, are characterized as bridge builders, and are able to overcome the obstacles posed by hierarchical structures.

Shared leadership is based on the concept of empowerment. It recognizes the significance of informal as well as formal leadership to the success of any enterprise. It acknowledges that no one person can possibly possess all the knowledge or power needed to accomplish intended goals or outcomes within the organization. Self-directed work teams and shared governance epitomize the philosophy of shared leadership. Shared governance is also a key principle in ANCC's Magnet Recognition Program.

Servant leadership puts other people and their needs before the leader's self-interest. The person who chooses to serve may be called on to lead and in so doing may transform the lives of her or his followers.

ORGANIZATION AND STRUCTURE

People work and practice within formal organizations. For the most part, healthcare organizations remain relatively traditional in their hierarchical arrangements.

Theories

Organizational Theory

The classical principles of organizational structure include chain of command, unity of command, and span of control. In today's dynamic business environment, these principles are challenged in practice if not in theory.

- *Chain of command* implies that a line of command exists unbroken from the top to the bottom of the organization. Each unit within the organization is connected to another. Hypothetically, reporting relationships are constrained, with each subsequent "layer" reporting administratively to the one immediately above it. In a positive sense, the chain of command ensures a smooth exchange of information from top to bottom and vice versa. In practice, however, the feedback loops necessary to ensure that upward as well as downward messages are heard and understood are at times absent.
- *Unity of command* holds that each subordinate is accountable to only one superior. Expectations are clearly defined and well understood.

- *Span of control* defines the scope of responsibility of a given supervisor or manager. Theoretically, tasks and responsibilities are divided so that goals are accomplished without undue burden on any one person or unit within the organization. Secondary to fiscal constraints in today's healthcare environment, the vast majority of managers' unity of command and span of control has expanded as healthcare organizations continue to downsize the number of managers.
- *Organizational charts* reflect the principles noted above, with each person or unit connected to another, generally in a hierarchical fashion. The extent to which organizational charts reflect actual behavior within organizations is questionable. Nonetheless, organizational charts do clarify relationships between and among people and functions within organizations and can be used to profile a variety of organizational structures. Organizational charts show formal relationships but not informal or informational connections among people or groups in organizations. Thus, they may show structure as it is assumed to be, not as it is. Organizational charts are labeled to illustrate how services are arranged within an establishment, such as service line (e.g., neurology, endocrinology, oncology), geography (e.g., 4 West, 4 South, 6 North), and service delivery (e.g., intensive care, transitional care, orthopedic surgery). Organizational charts also may reflect the manner in which the organization operates; in other words, provide a functional matrix.

Management Theory

Management, much like nursing, is considered both art and science. The "aim" of management is to create a surplus; that is, to establish an environment in which people can accomplish their goals with the least amount of time, money, materials, and personal dissatisfaction, or where they can achieve as much as possible of a desired goal with available resources.

Management came into its own in the 19th century, during the industrial age when guilds, crafts, and agriculture gave way to mass production and specialization. Management was and is seen as a means to accomplish an intended outcome through the work of others.

The traditional functions of management are as follows:

- *Plan:* Decide in advance what to do, how to do it, when to do it, and who is to do it.
- *Organize:* Establish an intentional structure of roles; assume that all tasks necessary to accomplish goals are assigned to people who can perform the tasks.
- *Staff:* Fill positions, and keep them filled.
- *Lead:* Influence people so that they willingly and enthusiastically work to achieve the goals of the organization.
- *Control:* Measure and correct activities of subordinates to ensure conformance to plans.
- *Coordinate:* Achieve harmony of individual efforts to achieve intended goals.

Scientific Management

Mechanical engineer Fredrick Taylor is considered the "father of scientific management." His era spans the late 19th and early 20th centuries and the beginning of the industrial age. Contemporaries include industrial engineer Frank Gilbreth; industrial and organizational psychologist Lillian Gilbreth; and mechanical engineers Henry Gantt, Harrington Emerson, and Morris Cook.

The major concept underlying the work of Taylor and his colleagues is that of efficiency. Efficiencies were created through the establishment of standards, time–motion studies, task analysis, job simplification, and productivity incentives.

Process Management

Mining engineer Henri Fayol is the champion of the management process school that came into vogue following World War I and during the Great Depression (early 20th century into the 1930s). Others whose work is associated with this era include social scientist Max Weber, anthropologist James Mooney, and business consultant Lyndall Urwick.

The process school examined the whole of an organization, not merely its parts. Competency rather than favoritism was seen as a driver of organizational management. Rules were established to govern practice, and workers could expect to be adequately compensated. Administratively, hierarchy prevailed, with clear delineation of one's authority based on the assigned position within the organization's traditional pyramidal structure. Authority to direct the activities of others flowed downward level by level. The "universal" principles of management—span of control, chain of command, accountability, responsibility, planning, organizing, coordinating, and controlling—were defined during this era.

Communication

One can compare communication to blood circulation in the human body. Just as blood is necessary to maintain life, communication is essential to maintain organizational life. Deprived of blood and therefore oxygen, cells malfunction and die. Deprived of necessary communication, individuals and departments within organizations malfunction. Research evidence suggests that accurate, relevant information in appropriate quantities improves decision-making and other kinds of performance for both individuals and groups.

Familiar managerial roles include planning, leading, directing, organizing, and controlling. In addition to formal authority, managers also have interpersonal roles, such as a figurehead, leader, and liaison. They have informational roles as monitor, disseminator, and spokesperson. And they have decision-making roles that include being an entrepreneur, intrapreneur, disturbance handler, resource allocator, and negotiator. The manager's position is endowed with status and authority by the organization because it is critical to a network of interpersonal relationships. In the interpersonal role, the manager is a figurehead (e.g., presenting awards). The goal of the manager is to accomplish the tasks and goals of the organization. The manager also will function in a communicator role as a liaison, as well as in an information role to obtain information on daily operations and disseminate necessary information to others to meet the goals of the organization. Managers are also the spokespersons representing their respective units of operation in management meetings. In the decision-making role, the manager is often a disturbance handler who deals with controversies that exist within the organization. The manager is a resource allocator, parceling out limited time, money, materials, and talent to best meet the organization's goals. Managers are also negotiators, who deal with on-the-spot bargaining and exchanging of information. What prevails in each of these roles is communication. Many studies have documented that managers spend the majority of their time communicating with others to fulfill their functions within the organization.

Some of the key principles of communication include active listening, reflective communication, two-way communication, and interviewing. Dr. Stephen Covey, in his book *Seven Habits of Highly Effective People*, lists communication as the fifth habit (Covey, 1989). Dr. Covey emphasizes that one first should attempt to understand what the other party is relaying prior to striving to be understood. When the sender transmits a message to the receiver, if the receiver does not clearly understand the message, the receiver should seek to clarify with the sender what the sender's exact meaning is. Communication occurs both verbally and nonverbally. Verbal communication involves speaking to another in a language that both parties understand. Nonverbal communication methods include body language, eye contact, and active listening. One of the problems with Internet and email communication is that nonverbal communication cannot be assessed.

There are three major characteristics associated with managerial communication: upward communication, downward communication, and lateral or diagonal communication. *Upward communication* carries information, such as work progress and news of problems for decision-making, to the manager. This communication comes from the subordinate and this information often is filtered. *Downward communication* flows from the manager to the subordinate to inform, direct, and control work activities, and also may be filtered. *Lateral or diagonal communication* occurs across the organization and between departments. This form of communication is used primarily for coordination and problem-solving, and occupies a great deal of time. Lateral or diagonal communication is a challenge because it involves intergroup relationships, is irregular, can interfere with daily routines, happens frequently and mushrooms in quantity quickly, and often involves ambiguous relationships. Networks of lateral communication are thus unstable, so a significant element in the art of managing is knowing the shifts in importance of information and acquiring, sharing, and making effective decisional use of that information.

There are six key processes in communication: thinking, encoding, transmitting the signal, perceiving, decoding, and understanding. *Thinking* involves framing the idea or message in the sender's mind; this is where the message is created. *Encoding* is placing the thought in some communicative form, such as speech or writing. *Transmitting* the signal is the actual sending of the message via some medium. These three areas of communication are done by the sender, but there must be a receiver of the message for communication to occur. The receiver must *perceive* the incoming communication with one or more senses (sight, hearing, feeling, taste, and smell). The receiver must *decode* the incoming communication into an understandable form. Finally, if the communication is successful, the receiver *understands* the message as it was intended to be understood by the sender. Given that all six processes must be performed successfully for communication to be effective, one can see how miscommunication can result if even one step in the communication process goes awry.

In addition to transmission of information, other types of communication include persuasive, assertive, aggressive, and passive-aggressive communication. The manager's role is often to persuade others to perform the task that needs to be accomplished. Persuasive communication prevails in such situations. Most managers use assertive communication, which always begins with the term "I" and not "you." The person using assertive communication speaks about him- or herself. For example, a person using an assertive style of communication would say "I am upset by that remark" rather than "You upset me." In the second example, the person is communicating aggressively, blaming the other person for his or her own feeling and thereby placing that other person in a defensive posture, which hinders the communication process. Passive-aggressive communication creates tension in an organization by expressing negative feelings in an indirect rather than a direct way. This apparently passive posture accomplishes the person's primary intention, so the person is actually being aggressive through use of a passive style of communication. An example would be a staff member who agrees or reports satisfaction with a manager's decision on a particular task, but actually disagrees with or resents the decision and therefore does not complete that task.

Some complications of communication include mismatches in meaning created by senders and receivers and lack of clarity in the values involved, which often result in unintended communication that creates disturbances. Barriers to communication include lack of congruence, distorted perceptions, distorted sources of information, defensive posture and behavior, and distortions from the past. Communication climates should be supportive, descriptive, problem-oriented, spontaneous, and empathetic, and should demonstrate equality and professionalism. Communication must above all be honest. Honest communication creates an environment of trustworthiness and credibility.

Another issue that can affect communication is our nation's cultural diversity, which means that to communicate effectively, one must be sensitive to different cultures. Cultural differences can affect both verbal and nonverbal communication. Consideration of generational diversity is also critical in the American workplace, which may include staff and managers from multiple generations. For example, a manner of communication that one generation deems respectful may be considered rude or stiff by another. Technology also affects communication. Email is eminently useful; however, the parties involved cannot see the nonverbal side of the communication process, which often results in miscommunicated messages that upset the receiver. It is important not to read emotion into email messages because this can contribute to a negative response.

The Institute of Medicine has documented that major quality problems often result from poor or incorrect communication. Many efforts have been made to avoid poor communication that results in poor quality patient care. SBAR (situation, background, assessment, recommendation) is one example of such efforts to ensure effective communication during patient handoffs or handovers. Documentation of patient care, whether through paper or electronic health records (EHRs), is a critical form of communication. Some problems with EHRs include boilerplate segments that fail to communicate a patient's particular situation and occasional documentation of care (often via checkbox) that has not really been rendered.

It is important to select the appropriate communication method for the target audience and the situation at hand. Examples of the methods available include email messages; role-playing; formal presentations; reports; communication at staff meetings; board meetings; one-on-one conversations; communication through a patient, family, or resident council; and consumer feedback. The appropriate communication message must be chosen for the respective audience and facility. For example, in a long-term-care setting, clients are residents and there is a resident council that provides consumer feedback to the facility on how to improve the facility, which serves as the residents' home. Many hospitals have initiated consumer advisory boards to advise the facility on care activities and services that are rendered or need to be rendered.

In summary, communication is the heart of management and leadership. Communication can make or break an organization. Good communication can contribute to positive patient care outcomes. Communication is much more than merely sending and receiving information; thought transmission and perception is at the crux of the matter.

Emotional Intelligence

Mayer and Salovey (1990) define *emotional intelligence* as:

> The ability to monitor one's own and others' feelings and emotions; to discriminate among them and to use this information to guide one's thinking and actions. (p. 20)

According to some, it is more important for a leader to have higher emotional intelligence than a high IQ.

There are models for emotional intelligence. For example, the Ability-Based Model for Emotional Intelligence views emotions as useful sources of information that help an individual make sense of and navigate the social environment. The model has several elements:

- *Perceiving emotions:* The ability to detect and decipher emotions in faces, pictures, voices, and cultural artifacts, and to identify one's own emotions. Perceiving emotions represents a basic aspect of emotional intelligence that makes all other processing of emotional information possible.
- *Understanding emotions:* The ability to comprehend emotional language and to appreciate complicated relationships that exist among emotions.
- *Managing emotions:* The ability to regulate emotions in ourselves and in others.
- *Using emotions:* The ability to harness emotions, even negative ones, and manage them to achieve intended goals and facilitate cognitive activities, such as thinking and problem-solving. The emotionally intelligent person can capitalize fully upon his or her changing moods to best fit the task at hand.

Understanding emotional intelligence is key when managing complex organizations.

Human Relations Management

The 1940s were a time of relative prosperity in the United States. Middle-class values predominated, the working class became more educated, and managers were able to focus attention on interpersonal relationships within the workplace. Harvard researchers George Elton Mayo, a psychologist, and Fritz Roethlisberger, a social scientist, conducted the Hawthorne Shirt Factory studies during this time. The Western Electric Company wanted to investigate the influence of working conditions on employee efficiency and productivity.

Although working conditions, specifically the level of light, were manipulated as part of the research design, the investigators found no correlation between workers' productivity and the condition of the environment. They did conclude that workers performed differently when they were being observed. Even today, the "Hawthorne effect" is frequently cited to explain the significance of relationships between managers and frontline workers relative to business outcomes, either positive or negative. While the validity and reliability of the Hawthorne study itself can be called into question, the term has taken its place in the management lexicon. Cooperation between labor and management, democratization of the workplace (in contrast to autocracy), and the criticality of communication are among the concepts that define this period.

Behavioral Science and Management

Psychologists Abraham Maslow and Fredrick Herzberg are associated with the behavioral school that gained prominence in the 1950s. Social psychologist Douglas MacGregor, social scientist Chris Argyris, organizational psychologist Rensis Likert, management theoretician Robert Blake, mathematician Jane Mouton, behavioral scientist Paul Hersey, industrial and organizational psychologist Fred Fiedler, and management consultant Kenneth Blanchard also gained distinction during this time. Their names and their work are likely to be familiar to many readers of this study guide. Indeed, several of their writings are considered management classics, and some have found a place in popular literature as well as in the academic arena. The One-Minute Manager (Blanchard & Johnson, 1982) and related spin-offs come to mind.

The behaviorists built on the work begun during the "human relations" period. Concepts that took shape during this time include:

- *Hierarchy of needs* holds that the needs of one level must be satisfied before a person can begin to satisfy the needs of the next level.
- *Personal motivators* and hygiene factors are complementary and equally important.
- *Workers need to have a say* in operations; self-direction results in satisfaction.
- *Leadership style* is important; participative management is the preferred mode.

The workforce during this era was relatively homogenous, fairly prosperous, and better educated. More women assumed jobs outside the home than traditional role responsibilities. Many women entered the workforce as a matter of national necessity during World War II; some stayed on after the war, although in jobs different than those they held during the 1940s.

Performance Improvement (PI)/Organizational Improvement (OI)

W. Edwards Deming, Joseph Juran, and Philip Crosby are the recognized leaders in the total quality management (TQM) and continuous quality improvement (CQI) arena. Although Deming's and Juran's work progressed quietly during the post–World War II years, it was conducted mostly in Japan. TQM and CQI did not gain popularity in the United States until the 1980s and 1990s in the wake of the realization that merchandise produced in Japan was often superior to and less expensive than goods produced elsewhere, including the United States. Examined more closely, the principles that underlie TQM and CQI are those of the scientific method conveyed in ways that generated acceptance by business leaders in the United States.

Deming's (2000) holistic approach maintains that the interaction of materials, machines, and people determines productivity, quality, and competitive advantage. Deming's 14 points (Deming, 2000) further articulate the foundation of TQM:

1. Create constancy of purpose; strive for long-term improvements rather than short-term profit.
2. Adopt the new philosophy; do not tolerate delays and mistakes.
3. Cease dependence on mass inspection; build quality into the process on the front end.
4. End the practice of awarding business on price alone; build long-term relationships.
5. Improve constantly and forever the system of production and service at each stage.
6. Institute training and retraining; continually update methods and thinking.
7. Institute leadership; provide resources needed for effectiveness.
8. Drive out fear; people must believe it is safe to report problems or to ask for help.
9. Break down barriers between departments; promote teamwork.
10. Eliminate slogans, exhortations, and arbitrary targets; supply methods, not buzzwords.
11. Eliminate numerical quotas; they are contrary to the idea of continuous improvement.
12. Remove barriers to pride in workmanship; allow autonomy and spontaneity.
13. Institute a vigorous program of education and retraining; people are assets, not commodities.
14. Take action to accomplish the transformation; provide a structure that enables quality.

The contributions of Walter Shewhart, the "father of statistical quality control," are sometimes overlooked in the popularization of TQM and CQI. Shewhart successfully brought together the disciplines of statistics, engineering, and economics and became known as the "father of modern quality control." The lasting and tangible evidence of that union—for which he is most widely known—is the simple but highly effective tool known as the *control chart*.

"Systems thinking," popularized by Peter Senge and his colleagues from Massachusetts Institute of Technology in *The Fifth Discipline* (Senge, 1990), grew out of the TQM and CQI movement. These concepts have moved into the healthcare realm under the guidance of physicians Donald Berwick and Paul Batalden and the Institute for Healthcare Improvement (IHI).

The Joint Commission on the Accreditation of Health Care Organizations (JCAHO, now The Joint Commission) adopted TQM and CQI and has built the principles into its requirements. Concepts that form the foundation of TQM and CQI include:

- Benchmarking,
- Statistical process control,
- Reduction of variation,
- Application of the Pareto Principle (i.e., focus on the "vital few" rather than the "trivial many"),
- Application of the plan–do–check–act (PDCA) cycle to achieve systems improvement,
- Systems modification in contrast to personal blame,
- Use of teams, and
- Focus on meeting customer needs.

Over time, the manager's role has changed from that of overseer and controller to one of coach and supporter. Characteristics of the modern manager include:

- The belief that people are basically "good" (trustworthy) and capable of change,
- Appreciation of the value of diversity in contrast to homogeneity,
- Awareness that power shared is power gained,
- Creative use of conflict in contrast to avoidance of dissension at all cost,
- Risk-taking in contrast to risk aversion, and
- Fostering collaboration rather than competition (particularly among staff who must work together to get the job done).

Today, most organizations use the term *performance improvement*. Healthcare organizations employ the use of different systems for monitoring performance improvement, such as the American Nurses Association's National Database of Nursing Quality Indicators (NDNQI) system, Lean Sigma Six, and Plane Tree.

Reimbursement is also tied to performance improvement, and patient satisfaction scores have become come a key indicator tied to reimbursement.

Nursing and Nursing Theory

As with management, nursing has undergone changes throughout the years in response to societal needs and professional reasoning. The Great Depression, World War II, cyclic nursing shortages, and economics all have played a role in modifying nursing's pathway.

Prior to the late 1920s and early 1930s, nurses in the field of public health in particular enjoyed relative independence in practice and commanded respect within the medical community. Their basic education took place in an academic setting instead of in a hospital environment. With a background in epidemiology as well as in patient care, they were on the forefront of community-based care systems.

The anticipated trajectory was interrupted with the severe economic downturn of the Great Depression and cutbacks in funding for highly effective nurse-managed programs. Although academic programs in nursing survived, the recommendations of the Brown Report, issued in 1923 (Gebbie, 2009), were not adopted, and the primary learning environment for nurses became the hospital setting.

The early "modern" era of nursing found nursing students in what some might call a "servant role," in that nursing students provided much of the care to hospitalized patients in return for the clinical education and "room and board." The students were almost exclusively young women, newly graduated from high school, unmarried, and committed to a career of service.

When World War II loomed on the horizon, registered nurses (RNs) were called to serve in the military, leaving a noticeable gap in the workforce even as more people were being cared for in the hospital setting. To fill the gap, the "practical nurse" role came into being as a hypothetically temporary solution to that era's nursing shortage. An abbreviated curriculum was created to prepare practical nurses to assume designated bedside duties, thereby freeing the RNs remaining in the private sector to become overseers of care more than direct caregivers. Through the legislative process, practical nurses were eventually able to sit for an examination and become licensed as LPNs (licensed practical nurses) or LVNs (licensed vocational nurses).

The role of the nurse's aide also came into being during this time to fill the need for caregivers. Most nurse's aides learned their trade on the job. Over the years, more formal nurse's aide training programs have been developed and are generally offered through adult learning or vocational training programs.

As nursing has taken on an increasingly professional mantle, so, too, have models of care evolved. The common thread among all models is that of the nursing process. The elements of the nursing process are assessment, planning, intervention, and evaluation. In other words, this scientific process that follow a distinctive model also forms the basis for modern management.

Nursing theories generally fall into three categories, but types of nursing theory should incorporate the four key concepts—nurse, person, environment, and health—that constitute the meta paradigm for nursing theory.

The first type of nursing theory is conceptual models, which are very broad and abstract. The second type, grand theories, also tend to be broad and abstract and therefore difficult to apply in practice. The third type of nursing theory, middle-range theory, tends to be more grounded and applicable to practice. Use of nursing theories, particularly middle-range theories, are increasing among Magnet organizations because they tend to be more relevant than conceptual models or grand theories to nurses in practice.

Nursing theory is a relatively recent construct, with most theory development taking place in the 1960s, 1970s, and later. However, nursing historians and researchers acknowledge (Tomey & Alligood, 2006) that Florence Nightingale's *environmental factors* concept fits the definition of descriptive theory, addressing the impact of the environment on health/illness-related issues.

Nightingale held that nurses did not need to be fully versed in the disease model to fashion a therapeutic environment. Rather, she demonstrated that fresh air, light, cleanliness, adequate nutrition, and quietness fostered healing and wellness. Her assertions about the body's "reparative processes" provided her students with a way to think about their practice as a distinct entity and not merely as an extension of medicine. She also is credited with applying statistics to the field of health care well in advance of the era when such practice became common.

Nursing owes a debt of gratitude to a handful of nursing educators who took their master's and doctoral degrees in education from the University of Columbia Teachers' College and then became pioneers in the design of theory-based curricula for the field of nursing. Hildegard Peplau, Virginia Henderson, Lydia Hall, Faye Abdellah, Imogene King, Ernestine Wiedenbach, and Martha Rogers are among the early Columbia graduates whose names are associated with modern theories of nursing. In the mid-1970s, the National League for Nursing made theory-based nursing a requirement for accreditation.

Nursing theory continues to evolve, as does the definition of nursing. The most recent iteration of the definition, first published in 1980, is articulated in the 2003 edition of *Nursing's Social Policy Statement* (American Nurses Association [ANA], 2003): "*Nursing* is the prevention of illness; the alleviation of suffering; and the protection, promotion, and restoration of heath in the care of individuals, families, groups, communities, and populations" (p. 7). The statement reinforces the assertion that nursing practice embraces four essential components:

1. Attention to the full range of human experience,
2. Integration of objective and subjective phenomena,
3. Application of scientific knowledge, and
4. Provision of care that fosters health and healing.

Brief sketches of several theories of nursing that reinforce nursing's intent are presented below. The list is not all-inclusive.

The focus of Hildegard Peplau's 1952 work (as cited in her 1991 work) was on the interactive processes that form the basis of the nurse–client relationship. The nurse serves as resource, counselor, and surrogate. The relationship between client and nurse is progressive and overlapping and proceeds through these phases:

- Orientation,
- Identification,
- Explanation, and
- Resolution.

Virginia Henderson, as cited in Tomey and Alligod (2006), saw nursing as embracing the whole person and defined the practice as

> Assisting the individual, sick or well, in the performance of those activities contributing to health or its recovery (or to peaceful death) that he would perform unaided if he had the necessary strength, will, or knowledge. And to do this in such a way as to help him gain independence as rapidly as possible. (p. 102)

Consistent with her definition, Henderson described the role of the nurse as *substitutive* (doing for the person), *supplementary* (helping the person), or *complementary* (working with the person), with the goal of helping the person become as independent as possible. She categorized nursing functions into 14 components based on meeting human needs, for example, breathing, eating and drinking, elimination, worship, work, and so forth.

Like Henderson, Faye Abdellah (1960; as cited in Tomey & Alligod, 2006) defined nursing as meeting the needs of the whole person—physical, emotional, intellectual, social, and spiritual. The nurse assumes responsibility for the care of the family as well as that of the client (patient). She or he is a problem-solver and decision-maker and formulates a plan of care that includes five dimensions:

1. Comfort,
2. Hygiene and safety,
3. Physiological balance,
4. Psychological and social factors, and
5. Community and sociological factors.

Abdellah identified 21 nursing problems that, if addressed by the nurse, lead to improvement in the client's status.

Ida Orlando (1961; as cited in Tomey & Alligod, 2006) focused on the nurse's response to the immediate need of the client in a given situation. The situation is characterized by these three elements:

1. Client behavior,
2. Nurse reaction, and
3. Nurse actions.

Once the nurse identifies the client's need, she or he acts "automatically or deliberatively" to meet the need and, in so doing, reduces the distress experienced by the client.

Myra Levine (1973; as cited in Tomey & Alligod, 2006) saw the client as someone who interacts with and adapts to his or her environment. Conservation of energy is a primary concern, and it is nursing's role to assist the client to conserve her or his "resources" to promote health. Levine's four conservation principles of nursing are

1. Conservation of client energy,
2. Conservation of structural integrity,
3. Conservation of personal integrity, and
4. Conservation of social integrity.

Dorothy Johnson (1968; as cited in Tomey & Alligod, 2006) proposed that nursing's role is to relieve illness-induced stress so that the client is more easily able to regain equilibrium and proceed through recovery. The nurse focuses on seven areas of behavior (behavioral subsystems) and intervenes to reestablish balance in any or all of the systems under stress as a means of restoring health.

Martha Rogers (1970; as cited in Tomey & Alligod, 2006) took nursing's theoretical framework to a new level by asserting that the human organism is an energy field in a constant state of change, coexisting in the universe. In other words, human beings are part of the universe and, as such, influence and are influenced by the environment that surrounds them and of which they are an integral part. Rogers viewed nursing as "humanistic science" and focused on the research aspects of the field.

Dorothea Orem (1971; as cited in Tomey & Alligod, 2006) embraced a philosophy of self-care and theorized that nursing's role is to intervene when the client is unable to fulfill her or his biological, psychological, developmental, or social needs. The nurse is responsible for determining why a client is unable to meet her or his needs in the listed dimensions and then intervenes to help the client regain the ability to provide self-care in any or all dimensions.

Betty Neuman's (1972; as cited in Tomey & Alligod 2006) theory is based on a holistic perspective that sees human beings as part of an "open system;" they are in a state of constant adjustment as they interact with, adjust to, and are adjusted by the environment. Neuman identified three categories of stressors that disrupt the system:

1. *Intrapersonal:* Within the self,
2. *Interpersonal:* Occurring between persons, and
3. *Extrapersonal:* Occurring outside the person (e.g., financial stressors).

Because nursing is concerned with restoring balance, the nurse's role is one of "systems management." Nursing actions are seen as preventative and are categorized by level:

1. *Primary:* Identify risk factors and strengthen defenses,
2. *Secondary:* Strengthen internal defenses by identifying priorities and establishing treatment plans, and
3. *Tertiary:* Educate to prevent recurrence.

Sister Callista Roy's adaptation model (1976; as cited in Tomey & Alligod, 2006) with subsequent revision and expansion, holds that people are coextensive with their physical and social environments and that nursing's role is to enhance the well-being of the patient and, by extension, the well-being of the earth ("cosmic unity"). The nurse identifies those demands that are causing problems for the client, determines how well she or he is adapting to the demands, and provides care to help her or him adapt more successfully. Roy proposes that all persons must adapt to the following demands:

1. Meeting basic physiological needs,
2. Developing a positive self-concept,
3. Performing social roles, and
4. Achieving balance between dependence and independence.

Madeleine Leininger's (1978; as cited in Tomey & Alligod, 2006) transcultural theory identified caring as the central focus and unifying domain of nursing. Transcultural nursing focuses on comparative study and analysis of different cultures and subcultures throughout the world with respect to their caring interventions, health–illness values, and patterns of behavior. The outcome is the development of a body of knowledge, both scientific and humanistic, from which to derive culture-specific and culture-universal nursing care practices.

Jean Watson (1979; as cited in Tomey & Alligod, 2006) reiterated that nursing is concerned with health promotion, health restoration, and prevention of illness and that these ends are achieved through the integration of science and philosophy by nurses, whose interpersonal interventions are designed to meet human needs.

Kathy Kolcaba's (2002) comfort theory embraced a concept with a strong association to nursing. Nurses traditionally provide comfort to patients and their families through interventions that can be called *comfort measures*. The intentional comforting actions of nurses usually are comforting to patients.

Enhanced comfort, as an immediate desirable outcome of nursing care, is theoretically and positively correlated with desirable health-seeking behaviors (HSBs). HSBs can be internal (e.g., healing, immune function, number of T cells), external (e.g., health-related activities, functional outcomes, hospital length of stay, hospital readmissions), or a peaceful death. The relationship between comfort and HSBs are clarified in Kolcaba's comfort theory.

Change Theory

Psychologists Abraham Maslow, Kurt Lewin, and Frederick Herzberg are associated with the motivational theories that underlie popularly referenced change models. Maslow's hierarchy of needs and Herzberg's two-factor theory are contrasted in Figure 2–1.

FIGURE 2–1.
MASLOW'S AND HERZBERG'S MOTIVATIONAL THEORIES

Hierarchy of Needs Theory		Two-Factor Theory
Self-actualization	Motivators	• Challenging work • Achievement • Growth in job • Responsibility
Esteem of status	Motivators	• Advancement • Recognition • Status
Affiliation or acceptance	Maintenance Factors	• Interpersonal relations • Company policy and administration • Quality of supervision
Security or safety	Maintenance Factors	• Quality of supervision • Working conditions • Job security
Physiological needs	Maintenance Factors	• Salary • Personal life

Adapted from *Organizational Behavior* (10th ed.), by J. R. Schermerhorn, J. Hunt, and R. N. Osborn, 2008, Hoboken, NJ: John Wiley & Sons. Copyright 2008 by John Wiley & Sons. Adapted with permission.

Lewin proposed that one maintains the status quo or a state of equilibrium by balancing both driving and restraining forces operating within any field. He maintained that, for any change to occur, this balance must be disrupted. One must either increase the power of the driving forces or lessen the power of the restraining forces. Conventional wisdom holds that it is generally easier or more productive to decrease the power of the restraining force, to decrease resistance, than to strengthen the driving forces. Lewin also suggested that the steps in the change process—unfreezing, movement, and refreezing—are predictable. Components associated with Lewin's phases of change include:

- Unfreezing
    - Gather data.
    - Diagnose the problem.
    - Decide if there is a need for change.
    - Make others aware of the need.
    - Confirm motivation for the change.
    - Proceed to movement only after the status quo has been sufficiently disrupted and others perceive the need for change.
- Movement
    - Develop a plan.
    - Set goals and objectives.
    - Identify areas of support and resistance.
    - Include all who will be affected by the change in planning for the change.
    - Set target dates.
    - Develop change strategies.
    - Implement change.
    - Support and encourage others through the change.
    - Use tactics designed to overcome resistance.
    - Evaluate the change.
    - Modify the change if necessary.
- Refreezing
    - Integrate change into the structure of the organization.
    - Put support in place to sustain the change.

Sociologist Everett Rogers's research regarding the diffusion of innovation deserves mention in any discussion about change. Here, greatly simplified, are a few of Rogers's concepts:

- Innovations that are perceived as having greater relative advantage and less complexity will be adopted more rapidly than other innovations.
- Adopter categories can be defined on the basis of innovativeness and more or less fall into a bell-shaped curve:
    - *Innovators (2.5%):* These risk-takers are adventurous, independent, constantly seeking information, and generally have the means (e.g., finances, connections) to be "out in front." The opinions of others are not particularly relevant.
    - *Early adopters (13.5%):* These pioneers translate the innovator's message for the early majority. They establish momentum for change and are respected opinion leaders.
    - *Early majority (34%):* These people are deliberate and adopt new ideas just before the average member of a system. They do not seek information on their own but are willing to hear and act on the message from the early adopters.
    - *Late majority (34%):* These people are skeptical and adopt new ideas just after the average member of a system. They respond to the pressure of peers and then change accordingly. Their restraint is important in the change process because it provides a provocative voice that sometimes moderates the rate of change or influences the change agents to use alternative tactics.
    - *Resistors (16%):* These people are traditional and the last in a social system to adopt an innovation; they pay little attention to the opinions of others. Their dissident voice is valuable in any major change effort. Resistors encourage taking a closer look prior to implementing a change or innovation and cause others to take a second look at the who, what, where, and why of doing something.

To understand the practical application of Rogers' work, one need only look at the adoption of the Internet as an accepted way of doing business, gathering information, or learning.

The rapidity with which change is adopted and sustained in an organization has much to do with leadership's understanding of the complexity of the change process. Only if the actual or perceived threat is of such magnitude that maintaining the status quo is tantamount to disaster can massive change occur quickly and throughout an entire organization. Even then, there will be some who find it impossible to change. In many cases, these people will leave or be asked to leave the organization. Lim and O'Connor (1995) call the need for large-scale change in the midst of crisis the "burning platform" scenario.

Decision-Making

The "rational" model of decision-making in organizations is no longer considered the only option. A concept called *bounded reality* is probably more reasonable because the assumptions of the rational model rarely hold true in organizational life. *Bounded reality*, a term coined by Nobel laureate Herbert Simon (Bateman & Snell, 2002), holds that leaders in organizations cannot make perfectly rational decisions because

1. They have imperfect and incomplete information about alternatives and consequences,
2. They face highly complex problems,
3. They cannot process all the information that confronts them (human capacity),
4. They do not have sufficient time to fully process the information that confronts them, and
5. They are faced with conflicting goals among the constituents of the organization.

Systems Theory

The theoretical construct underlying systems holds that systems are composed of interrelated parts and that the arrangement of these parts results in a unified whole. Systems can be closed or open. *Closed systems* are assumed to occur only in the physical sciences (e.g., the circulatory system). *Open systems* interact internally and with the environment.

Organizations are defined as complex, sociotechnical open systems. Parts of the system are labeled as input, throughput, and output. *Input* is composed of such elements as staff, patients, materials, financial resources, supplies, and equipment. *Throughput* is the *process* that is performed to create a product. *Output* is the *product*; within the healthcare system, it may be defined as restored health, dignified death, research, education, and so forth.

While systems theory provides a useful language to describe organizational operations, it falls short when attempting to identify, let alone describe, the numerous variables at work throughout the input–process–output (IPO) process (Schermerhorn et al., 2002).

MISSION AND PHILOSOPHY

Purpose

The *mission statement* of an organization provides a general statement about its reason for *existence*, or its *purpose*. Its *vision statement* describes its *aspiration(s)*, the goal(s) it wishes to achieve. The mission and vision statements of an organization are meant to inspire and motivate those associated with it. Both are relatively brief and must be developed before the goals, objectives, and strategies of the establishment can be derived from them.

The mission statement flows from the organization's foundations. Does the organization have a social or community commitment? Does it have an educational affiliation? Whom does it exist to serve? What is the scope of services it provides?

Mission statements are future-oriented and speak to what an organization intends to achieve, given the resources at its disposal. Although idealistic, mission statements are created with the belief that what is promised is indeed attainable by the organization. Whether an organization's mission statement serves as an inspiration has more to do with how well and how consistently the people in the organization, particularly those who hold positions with the greatest power, act in ways that demonstrate their commitment to the organization's mission. Mission statements often are created at the higher echelons of organizations and may or may not reflect the beliefs and practices of those who work at the operational level.

Progressive organizations in which contemporary management exists generally have more defined and more comprehensive mission statements. The best statements involve staff as well as administration in the process of defining what the mission of the organization really is. Organizations that embrace this philosophy generally experience profound growth as employees truly understand as well as implement the mission.

Organizational Concepts and Models

Organizations can be structured in a variety of ways.

- *Vertical integration* provides different but complementary services among the parties involved (e.g., the affiliation of a particular hospital with a health maintenance organization).
- *Horizontal integration* indicates shared or reciprocal services across two or more institutions (e.g., the provision of cardiac surgical services by one affiliate and the provision of oncology services by another).

- In a *joint venture*, one partner provides a needed service while the other partner ensures its financing.
- Organizations or units within organizations may be structured by function or by product line. In a *functional* model, decision-making is centralized and coordination among groups or entities may be lacking. A *matrix* structure integrates functions and products and by its very nature may "violate" the unity-of-command principle because those who operate within this structure may have complex reporting relationships.
- *Shared governance* fosters ownership of the work to be done by formally involving those who perform it in decisions about structure, performance, staffing, and resource allocation.

Framework

The mission and vision of an organization are consistent with the organization's structural intent. For example, the mission statement for a small rural community hospital that provides a few primary care services will reflect that reality, and its text will differ considerably from the mission statement of the huge academic tertiary center in a metropolitan area 50 miles away. The intent of both is to offer accurate statements consistent with their particular aspirations, not to hold themselves out as something they are not.

The mission statements of academic health centers deserve special mention. The reason that many academic institutions devoted to health care exist is to provide a learning environment for practitioners in the early phase of their careers and to perform health-related research. The "caring language" characteristic of the mission statements of many community hospitals, even of those that are quite large or part of multihospital systems, may be missing from the mission statements of some academic institutions. Patient care may be listed as a secondary purpose.

This distinction is important because those who seek employment in any organization should do their best to ensure that their personal and professional values are aligned with those of the institution before accepting a job offer.

Format

The mission and the vision statements are meant to instill confidence in those who seek care from the institution and pride in those who practice within its walls. They should be appealing in appearance, clear in their wording, understandable to the community at large, and easily recalled by the organization's staff.

Review Mechanisms

Mission and vision statements undergo periodic review to ensure consistency with actual practice. In general, the mission, vision, and philosophy of an organization are carefully reviewed as part of the episodic accreditation process, whether through the Joint Commission or some other accrediting body.

PLANNING CONTINUUM

The planning process includes the following steps:

1. Performing assessments,
2. Setting goals,
3. Establishing objectives (plans), and
4. Determining actions.

Planning addresses the who, why, what, when, where, and how an organization will function to achieve its intended objectives.

Strategic Planning

Strategic planning involves defining the long-term objectives of the organization and setting priorities. The timeline is future-oriented and predicts organizational activities over several years. The capital building plan is an example of strategic planning.

Assessment

Assessment implies determining the strengths, weaknesses, opportunities, and threats (SWOT) that face the organization, analyzing risks, determining the preferred future state, and securing potential resources

Goal Setting

Strategic goals set the organization's path for several years into the future. The more the goals are consistent with the vision and values of the organization and are well defined, the greater the likelihood they will be achieved, absent unanticipated crises.

Prioritizing

Because there is always the possibility that a reversal of fortune could occur, organizations need to set priorities and get critical buy-ins from key stakeholders during the planning process. Dependencies need to be considered when establishing priorities to avoid unexpected surprises.

Evaluation

Measures of success must be established at the outset so that the anticipated outcome of any strategic initiative is known in advance and can be measured on an ongoing basis.

Contingency Planning

Contingency planning involves managing the business in the moment and determining proactively what is to be done during unexpected occurrences. In many ways, contingency planning is the way businesses operate on a day-to-day basis.

Program Planning

Program planning considers the organization's capacity to successfully execute a particular plan or service. Programs selected by the organization must match its overall philosophy, be financially sound, and in general create a profit for the organization. Some programs may be mandated (e.g., mental health services in a health maintenance organization) or voluntary (e.g., a full-scope, freestanding women's health service).

HEALTHCARE ENVIRONMENT

PRACTICE ENVIRONMENT

Nursing Care Delivery Systems and Professional Practice Models

Briefly described below are several models of practice that have been embraced within the field of nursing over the years.

- *Functional nursing:* Required tasks are divided among staff, with each nurse taking responsibility for executing an assigned function (e.g., "IV nurse," "dressing nurse," "procedure nurse"). This approach is not unlike the industrial model used in other segments of the business world.
- *Team nursing:* Required care for a group of patients is carried out by several team members, such as the RN, LPN, nurse's aide, and physical therapy aide. The RN serves in the role of team leader, and as such, has the opportunity to apply managerial skills as a means of accomplishing the work at hand.
- *Primary nursing:* The responsibility for the care of the patient, or group of patients, rests exclusively with the RN. Primary nursing has been interpreted in a variety of ways: (1) the RN provides all care for the patient during her or his shift of duty; (2) the "primary" RN assumes 24-hour accountability for the care of the patient, with "associates" overseeing the patient's care when the primary care RN is not in attendance; or (3) while the nurse is the primary caregiver and cannot delegate authority, she or he is assisted by others in the provision of direct care while maintaining overall responsibility for the patient. The core elements of primary nursing include continuity of care for the patient; accountability of the nurse for the patient's care; care that is comprehensive, individualized, and coordinated; and the professional satisfaction of the nurse.
- *Total patient care:* This mode of practice is akin to the first approach described under primary nursing. The RN cares exclusively for one or a small group of patients. This mode of practice is common in specialty services such as intensive care.
- *Relationship-based care:* Relationships are established with the patient. The goal is to work collaboratively with the patient to effect a positive outcome.
- *Transforming care at the bedside:* The goal is to empower nursing to improve care delivery and the outcomes of care at the bedside by identifying initiatives for quality improvement.

An example would be improving medication delivery through a computerized medication administration system, such as bar-coding.

- *Family-centered care:* The goal is to care for not only the patient but also the family by including the family in all aspects of care as the patient permits. Note that "family" has different meanings for different patients (e.g., a significant other not legally related may be the patient's family).
- *Synergy model of patient care:* This is the preferred model for patient care developed by the American Association of Critical Care Nurses (AACN). Elements of the model include:
  - Needs of the patient are at the core of this model.
  - The needs of the patient are matched to the competencies of the nurse. This is a critical element of this model.
  - The ideal relationship is one that is characterized by the patient moving safely through the healthcare delivery system.

Collaborative Practice

Collaborative practice takes place when members of various disciplines, each with a particular set of skills needed by the patient or family, come together to plan and deliver care. The term initially came into use as intentional collaboration between the disciplines of nursing and medicine was being formalized.

Other Models

- *Ambulatory care:* Primary care, clinics, private offices, federally qualified health centers
- *Assisted living facilities:* Services for the elderly and others requiring assisted care in a supervised manner are provided in an apartment-like environment, where the resident is more or less self-sufficient. Residents can dine in a main dining room. Many facilities that provide comprehensive services have independent apartments, assisted living, and traditional long-term-care services as a continuum of care.
- *Home health:* Governed by the OASIS Program of the Centers for Medicare and Medicaid Services
- *Long-term care:* Care of elderly and others, such as subacute and rehabilitation care, as well as traditional nursing home care. A noted change is occurring in long-term care. The term "nursing home" is not used that frequently today; many long-term-care facilities use the term "health center" to designate the subacute services rendered in nursing homes.
- *Rehabilitation care:* Service offered by long-term-care facilities, physical rehabilitation centers, and residential care centers

Differentiated Practice and Case Management

In this model, the care delivered is based on the educational level and expertise of the nurses who assume responsibility for one or more patients. For example, a clinical nurse specialist, an RN, and an LPN each may contribute to the patient's care and collaborate in such a way that each brings her or his particular skills to bear in ensuring that the patient receives needed care. In another sense, differentiated nursing care defines specialization (e.g., renal nursing, burn unit nursing, ambulatory care nursing).

In differentiated nursing care and case management, the RN is placed in the position of effectively managing the care of a group of patients as they move through the continuum of care, perhaps from the inpatient setting, to the convalescent setting, to the home with the assistance of home care, and eventually to independence. Case management is a growing field for nurses in all settings.

Case managers coordinate needed care for a designated group of patients on the basis of defined characteristics of the group. Third-party payers may use case managers who are responsible for reviewing the cost and relative effectiveness of proposed care and recommending approval or denial of the requested intervention. They also may suggest alternative, less costly interventions. RNs constitute the largest group of case managers employed by insurance providers and work closely with the medical directors of these same plans.

Case or care managers also practice in healthcare organizations, where they coordinate care for various groups of patients, often by disease category (e.g., diabetes, asthma, heart failure). Case or care management is a growing field within nursing and is generally seen as a satisfying career choice.

Good research models for determining the effectiveness of case or care management are being developed and applied in the field. Despite empirical claims that the programs are effective, how effective they are is yet to be determined. Because of the nature of the population served, "true" cost savings may not be achieved, at least longitudinally. This possibility needs to be balanced against the probability that case management is the "right thing" to do, whether it significantly reduces costs.

Critical and Clinical Pathways

Clinical pathways define intended outcomes and provide direction for care. They are variously known as clinical practice guidelines, protocols, or critical paths and may apply to care provided in one setting (e.g., the hospital), or they may extend across the continuum of care. They are generally developed and intended for use by multidisciplinary teams and are evidence-based (i.e., the recommended actions are based on scientific studies to the extent such studies have been done). As with other such instruments, they follow the "law of averages," and variation must be explained or justified. Clinical pathways may be prescriptive (e.g., "Do it this way") or descriptive (e.g., "This is the recommendation").

The extent to which clinical pathways form the foundation for practice is as yet unknown. Even though such guidelines exist in all care settings, the degree of buy-in on the part of the various disciplines has not reached critical mass. Nonetheless, as regulatory agencies and quality oversight groups look more closely at variation in practice, the likelihood that clinical pathways will be implemented and followed increases.

While it may be a matter of semantics, the concept of critical path, as opposed to clinical path, may benefit by clarification. The term critical path, which is derived from the profit management literature, is set up in such a way that target timelines for critical elements are established. In addition, the steps along the path are sequential, with the beginning of the next step contingent on successful completion of the prior step. Software programs for critical path management are available.

Alternative Care Settings

The variety of settings in which nurses practice is broad and ever-expanding. The following are just a few of the options available to nurses whose practice extends beyond the hospital:

- Ambulatory care
- Rehabilitation centers
- Schools and student health services
- Industrial and corporate nursing
- Long-term care (LTC)
- Armed services
- Public health
- Research
- Nurse-managed community clinics
- Case management or utilization management within a managed care organization
- Parish nursing

Nurses have increasing opportunities to demonstrate their value in settings beyond the hospital. The extent to which nurses are perceived as contributors to the success of any endeavor, the better the public may come to understand the significant contribution that nurses make to the field of health care.

Governance Models

As with governance higher in the organizational structure, *unit-level governance* can take a variety of forms. In a traditional hierarchy, lead staff report to a charge nurse, who in turn reports to a nurse manager, who then reports to a unit manager or coordinator or assistant manager, and so on up the chain of command.

A newer model, that of *shared governance,* may be more successful in the long run. Shared governance allows staff nurses to be part of the decision-making process about the organization of work on their unit or service. For example, the 22 entities that make up the Seton Healthcare Network in Central Texas (see http://www.Seton.net) embrace shared governance. Seton has established a Nursing Practice Congress that meets monthly to "collectively set and evaluate nursing care standards across the Network" (Seton Healthcare Network, 2009). According to Seton's public relation's materials,

> Shared governance empowers frontline staff nurses to actively participate on policy-making bodies that determine the professional nursing practice environment at SETON. The integrity of the governance model relies upon meaningful participation of staff nurses—at meetings of staff, department Practice Councils, Specialty Councils, and the Nursing Congress. (Seton Healthcare Network, 2009)

Several of the network's facilities have been awarded ANCC Magnet Recognition status.

The assumed outcome of shared governance is greater accountability for practice, greater staff satisfaction, improved clinical outcomes, and greater efficiency. Labor–management partnerships in unionized environments strive for similar outcomes.

Corporate Culture and Climate

Corporate culture is characterized by a system of shared actions, values, and beliefs that develops within an organization and guides the behavior of its members. Corporate culture is a pervasive force, and its power is not always appreciated unless it is breached either intentionally or unintentionally.

Culture or climate helps those within the organization define the characteristics of their organization, helps those new to the organization to "fit in," and clarifies the organization to those outside its boundaries. Awareness of the organization's culture in advance of employment helps potential employees determine if their own values and those of the organization are in sync. If they are not, then the applicant may wish to seek employment with another company. Corporate culture can change, but it rarely does so in response to a single individual.

Those who observe such phenomena believe that cultural differences have a major impact on the performance of organizations and the quality of work life experienced by those within the organization.

Autocratic

The *autocratic* organization is generally perceived as a "top-down" entity, with decisions made at the executive level and then announced to the workforce. Managers and administrators are expected to enforce the decisions; thus, their efforts are directed toward helping staff accept decisions that have already been made. Techniques used to gain compliance include coercion, threats of punishment, and clear direction of actions.

While autocracy certainly has its detractors—and it is hardly a preferred practice in today's business environment—there may be times when an autocratic approach means the difference between success and failure of a business, particularly a business that finds itself in crisis with a very short window of opportunity for turnaround.

Bureaucratic

A *bureaucratic* culture is characterized by reliance on rules, regulations, policies, and procedures. While all organizations need practical policies and procedures to avoid chaos, rules are central to the bureaucratic organization. Proponents of the bureaucratic approach believe that personnel compliance with the norms of the organization can best be achieved through external motivation engendered by fear of reprisal if rules are broken. Some tout government agencies as the classical example of bureaucracy, even labeling staff members as *bureaucrats*. In reality, many bureaucratic organizations, healthcare institutions among them, exist outside of government, and many government agencies now operate in a more participative manner.

Participative

A *participative* culture is characterized by openness to input from all levels within the organization as part of the decision-making process. It is important to distinguish input from the actual *decisions* leaders must make. Employees are sometimes disappointed when the final decision is contrary to or significantly different from the suggestions they have given. In a participative culture, managers and administrators have an obligation to let employees know in advance how their input will be used.

Those who subscribe to a participative philosophy believe that employees are internally motivated to achieve the goals of the organization because their personal values are consistent with those of the organization. Employees respond more favorably to encouragement and coaching than to top-down direction, to rule-bound dictates, or to reprimand.

The term *situational* is sometimes used to describe the leadership style that may be seen in a participative culture. Here is a brief explanation of the continuum of options available to managers:

- *Decide:* Managers make a decision and may or may not receive input from individuals or groups before announcing that decision.
- *Consult individually:* Managers present a problem to group members individually, then obtain their input, and ultimately decide themselves.
- *Consult group:* Managers present a problem to the group as a whole, then obtain their input, and ultimately decide themselves.
- *Facilitate:* Managers present a problem to the group, set boundaries, facilitate the group but have no greater say in outcome than any other member of the group, and the group decides.
- *Delegate:* Managers set boundaries for the group, then step out of active participation in the work of the group and provide behind-the-scenes resources and encouragement; the group decides.

Clinical Advancement Program or Career Ladder

Clinical ladders foster recognition of clinically expert nurses and offer a career pathway that allows them to continue providing direct care to patients. In general, those who elect to "climb" the clinical ladder need to demonstrate their expertise through testimony of colleagues and supervisors and presentation of exemplars clearly detailing how their application of the nursing process has made a difference in the outcome of care for one or more clients. This process has been well outlined by Patricia Benner and her colleagues in the classic text *From Novice to Expert* (2001).

The career ladder may be seen somewhat differently; it suggests that the nurse will move intentionally through a career path that builds on and fosters development of her or his leadership skills—perhaps moving "through the ranks" from charge nurse to manager and eventually to an executive-level position—depending on skill, education, and availability of sponsorship and mentoring.

Consistent with ANA's standards of performance and practice for nursing administrators (ANA, 2004), those who desire to move into the administrative rank of nursing have an obligation to prepare themselves to do so both academically and experientially.

Alternatively, the nurse's career ladder may take a more clinical direction, moving from staff nurse to clinical nurse specialist or perhaps to nurse practitioner or educator.

Collaboration and Consultation

Collaboration implies that various parties, physicians and nurses in particular, engage in joint problem-solving with the best interest of the client(s) foremost in mind. In a management sense, collaboration means that the involved parties come together to solve the problem in an atmosphere of mutual respect. This approach is of particular value when the goals of both parties are too critical to be compromised.

Consultation occurs when the knowledge needed to better identify a problem rests outside the staff member's current realm or scope of practice. The consultant brings her or his expertise and objectivity to the problem-solving process. The person requesting the consultation recognizes her or his own limitations, gains valuable insight during the consultation process, and is then able to apply this learning in other situations. For example, the new nurse manager may request consultation with the corporate controller or with the financial analyst to better understand the budget process. In the clinical setting, the nurse new to the oncology clinic may request consultation with the highly experienced clinical nurse specialist in establishing a care plan for the patient with acute myelogenous leukemia undergoing experimental chemotherapy.

Integrated Healthcare System

In an integrated healthcare system (e.g., networks, consortia), providers agree to accept the risk of caring for a particular segment of the population for a pre-established fee and to provide needed care across the continuum in a cost-effective manner. Preventive care is inherent in this system, with primary care providers, not the hospital, at the center of the equation. Keeping people healthy is seen as a way to use resources most efficiently; therefore, decreasing the need for hospitalization is both the goal and outcome of the integrated healthcare system.

Systems may be *vertically* or *virtually integrated.* In *vertical integration*, hospitals, medical groups, and other delivery system elements are brought together under one umbrella with shared purpose and unity of control. Potential challenges include relatively high overhead and internal power struggles. In *virtual integration*, systems are linked contractually; purpose is shared, but control remains more or less autonomous. One challenge is that virtually integrated groups may remain committed to being a part of the system only to the extent that the new system is perceived as more advantageous than any other alternative.

For healthcare organizations that have their own "brand identity" to form a consortium with other organizations, the culture of each organization should be thoroughly assessed for compatibility. To leave relationships to chance or to automatically assume that greater integration will occur because of a pronouncement can prove disastrous.

INSTITUTIONAL ENVIRONMENT

Organizational Structure

Centralized vs. Decentralized

The *centralized* organization is a typical hierarchy that follows the traditional chain-of-command concept and is characterized by top-down decision-making. The more decision-making is "pushed down" the chain of command, the more *decentralized* the organization becomes. With increased decentralization, lower-level managers have more opportunity to develop their executive skills and achieve greater job satisfaction.

Product Line

Product line structure, structure by specialization, has several advantages: task assignments are clear and are related to employees' skills; employees can build on one another's knowledge, training, and experience; new managers have a ready-made laboratory in which to enhance their skills; and the product line is easy to explain.

Product lines can be further characterized as functional or divisional. The term *functional* is self-explanatory. For example, surgical oncology, head injury rehabilitation, and endocrinology can be characterized as functional product lines. *Divisional* product lines cluster products, services, clients, or legal entities in geographically dispersed areas with the intent of increasing market share. Critics of divisional dispersion suggest that duplication of effort and service may occur under this model, and thus, the hypothetical advantages of the product line may be compromised.

Matrix

Matrix organizations combine functional and divisional patterns and assign individuals to more than one unit. From the perspective of classic managerial theory, the matrix model defies the unity-of-command principle in that it requires employees to report to more than one "boss." In practical terms, and with the complexity of the modern workplace, the matrix organization makes sense and may occur *organically* (i.e., it will simply come into being because it works) or *purposely* (i.e., it will be intentionally created because of its value).

Exquisite communication is required for a matrix organization to succeed. In the absence of open, dynamic formal and informal communication links, the overlapping authority and responsibility of managers may lead to conflicts, gaps in productivity, and inconsistent practice.

Committee

A *committee* brings together a group of people with the intent of achieving a common task or goal. Committees may be formal or informal or permanent or *ad hoc* (convened for a short time for a particular purpose). An ad hoc committee may be termed a *task force*. The existence of certain committees is specified in the organization's bylaws and may be mandated by external regulatory agencies.

To the extent possible, committee size should be such that work can be accomplished consistent with principles of group formation and cohesiveness. Groups of 5 to 10 tend to accomplish their assigned tasks more efficiently than do larger groups. If the committee must be large to meet political or organizational intent, then the creation of *subcommittees* within the group may help the committee move its work forward more quickly.

Planning is key to committee success. In an ideal situation,

- The agenda should be well planned and published in advance.
- The committee should ideally create a charter for itself so that its intent and link to the larger organization are clear.
- Ground rules should be established early on.
- Meetings should start and end on time.
- Each meeting should have a stated purpose.
- Participants should come to the committee with their assignments complete and ready to participate fully in the work of the group.
- Opposing viewpoints should be welcomed and respected.
- The group should remain focused.
- Meaningful reports should be generated as a result of the committee's work.
- Time spent in committee meetings and in the accomplishment of committee tasks should further the goals of the organization.

Governing Boards

The *board of directors* of an organization makes major decisions affecting the organization. The board is led by a chairperson, governed by a set of bylaws, and responsible for discharging the following duties:

- Selecting, assessing, rewarding, and sometimes replacing the chief executive officer;
- Determining the strategic direction of the organization and reviewing its financial performance; and
- Ensuring that the activities of the organization are ethical, socially responsible, and legal.

Systems Integration

Networks

Networks allow entities to come together as a way of providing greater value to a community, consolidating power or market share, or enhancing fiscal solvency through collective purchasing power.

Network relationships allow for organizational autonomy on one hand and coalitional power on the other. For example, several hospitals in a particular geographical area may determine that it is in their best interest to form a coalition for the purpose of joint purchasing and contracting. However, each facility retains its independent internal system of governance.

The concept of network also applies to communications. Communication networks may be decentralized, centralized, or restricted. In a *decentralized* system, direct communication occurs up, down, across, in, and out without restriction. *Centralized* communication implies that input and output is controlled to a greater or lesser extent through a "hub" or control point. *Restricted* networks place intentional barriers between groups, particularly those that disagree with one another's positions. (One might suggest that the term *restricted network* is an oxymoron.)

Continuity of Care

Continuity of care implies that the services needed to promote the client's health and well-being are coordinated within and across the continuum of services provided in the outpatient, inpatient, rehabilitative, or continuing care setting and home care or hospice. At each point in the process, the patient's or family's preferences and values should be considered along with the needs and demands of the organization.

In the acute or extended care settings, discharge planners, generally nurses or social workers, play a key role in ensuring that the needs of the patient are anticipated at the next level of care to which she or he proceeds.

Well-orchestrated continuity of care ensures that patient needs are met in the most cost-effective manner possible. This ideal often is frustrated because of the fragmentation that characterizes the current healthcare system.

Restructuring

Organizations restructure in response to a variety of internal or external factors. Restructuring is seen as a means to reduce duplication of effort and to increase productivity. A caveat: The investment in restructuring to gain promised efficiencies needs to be examined carefully. Such scrutiny should occur before the initiation of restructuring efforts. However, the dubious investment in restructuring is sometimes identified only after the fact.

Internal

Internal restructuring refers to a change in communication channels, reporting relationships, functions of various business units or departments within an organization, or even job titles and duties.

External

External restructuring follows the decision to integrate disparate entities or in the presence of mergers or new affiliations. For example, two hospitals in close proximity to one another may elect to merge their establishments (provided, of course, that they meet any legal challenges encountered along the way). As a result of the merger, only one administrative team is needed, generally a combination of the two previously existing teams. Those whose positions are now redundant may be offered severance packages, or they may be offered other positions within the new organization.

EXTERNAL ENVIRONMENT

The healthcare system is not confined to hospitals or clinics. Rather, it is composed of a far-reaching network of affiliates, regulatory agencies, and special interest groups or organizations. In addition, the environment is influenced by healthcare access, the surrounding community, interagency relationships, the healthcare industry itself, and national and international factors.

Community Organizations

Community organizations exist to serve the needs of defined populations or to promote and garner resources for specific activities. Community clinics often are established to serve the needs of those with low incomes or who do not have health insurance. Government funding through defined allocations or grants, supplemented by private contributions often through foundations, constitutes the funding source for community clinics. For example, in 1999, the Tides Foundation established the Community Clinics Initiative in California to improve the technology and information systems of the state's nonprofit community clinics.

The American Red Cross, the American and Canadian Lung Associations, the Muscular Dystrophy Association, the American Diabetes Association, and the American Heart Association are but a few of the many examples of community organizations, many funded largely with donations from private citizens, that exist to provide a variety of services to those in need.

Access to Care

Access to care may be defined as the entry into or use of healthcare services. Access is generally seen as inseparable from cost and quality; that is, cost, quality, and access are generally addressed as the balancing forces that lead to improvement or disintegration of health, whether of an individual or of a community.

Paradoxically, increased access may in some cases actually decrease the cost of care, or lessened expenditures may improve the quality of care. For example, the person with diabetes who has access to early intervention and ongoing support through the healthcare system supplemented with involvement in a local diabetes association may stay in better control of the disease and avoid its devastating and costly cardiovascular and renal sequelae.

The dimensions of access include the following:

- *Geographical* access is affected by where people live in relation to where services are available. Someone living in a remote area of Alaska will not have the same geographic access to care as a person living in metropolitan Chicago.
- *Physical* access is influenced by the capability and mobility of people to reach the locations where care is provided.
- *Temporal* access refers to the match between the hours the healthcare system is available and the relative convenience of those hours to people who seek care.
- *Sociocultural* access refers to the match between expectations of a given cultural group and the ability of the healthcare system to meet those expectations.
- *Financial* access is mediated by the ability to pay for services provided. In the United States, most financial access to care is through third-party payers (i.e., insurance of one type or another).
- *The Affordable Care Act of 2010* is expected to improve access to care by offering an estimated 33 million more American citizens insurance coverage through insurance exchanges that begin implementation in 2014.

Community Assessment, Demographic Assessment, and Feasibility Studies

Studies are conducted to determine priority health needs and the gaps in services and systems required to meet those needs in a defined geographical location. Such studies measure the prevalence of chronic health conditions; the need and adequacy of mental health and substance abuse services; demographics and socioeconomic trends; and the need for and adequacy of acute care, long-term care (LTC), specialty care, and public health services. Findings then become the stimulus for initiatives and for community or professional education. Whether the studies are undertaken locally as a discreet task or by one of the many public policy institutes available for such activities depends on the scope, intent, and funding allocated for the study.

Community Diagnosis and Epidemiology

Epidemiology refers to the study of the prevalence of a disease or health condition and the factors that determine its prevalence. Protection of the public is implied and, as such, epidemiology is concerned with the health of populations rather than of individuals. *Descriptive epidemiology* considers time, place, and person. *Analytic epidemiology* is concerned with the agent, host, and environment and, as a matter of course, follows descriptive epidemiology.

Interagency Relationships

Various agencies involved with the delivery of health care are obligated to maintain relationships with one another. For example, hospitals are obligated to inform the Public Health Department about the occurrence of certain infectious diseases. The Centers for Medicare and Medicaid Services is obligated to inform care delivery systems of changes in reimbursement policies for care provided to Medicare and Medicaid recipients.

In a wholly integrated system—which the U.S. healthcare system is *not*—such relationships would likely be better defined than they are at present.

Healthcare Industry

The term *healthcare industry* refers to the conglomerate of products, people, and services involved with the delivery of health care in the United States.

- American health care is "big business"—a trillion-dollar industry. In 2008, the gross domestic product (GDP) devoted to health care–related expenditures was 17%, up from 8.8% in 1980, and grew to 17.9% by 2010 (Henry J. Kaiser Family Foundation, 2012). Total spending was $2.4 trillion in 2007, or $7,900 per American citizen. It is projected that healthcare expenditures will reach $4.3 trillion and that the percentage of GDP will reach 20% by 2016. In 2008, healthcare spending in the United States reached $2.4 trillion and was projected to reach $3.1 trillion by 2012 (Keehan et al., 2008).
- Analysts predict that the percentage of U.S. financial resources devoted to health care will continue to grow in the years ahead.

- Annual premiums that a health insurer charges an employer for a health plan covering a family of four averaged $12,700 in 2008. Employees contributed nearly $3,400, or 12% more than they did in 2007 (Henry J. Kaiser Family Foundation, 2008).

Driving forces for healthcare costs include pharmaceuticals, medical devices, and other medical advances; general inflation; rising provider expenses; government mandates and regulations; increased consumer demand; litigation and risk management; excessive administrative expenses; inflated prices; poor management and inappropriate care, waste, and fraud; and other factors such as a proposed national health plan for the nation's uninsured population. These problems significantly increase the cost of health care and health insurance for employers and workers.

National and International Factors

While the United States spends more per capita on health care than any other industrialized nation, the healthcare expenditures in other developed countries also are rising, regardless of system of care. This increase is fueled by factors similar to those identified above and, in particular, the changing demographics that show a significant rise in the number of elderly persons. The extent to which costs can be contained in the near term remains in question.

Other sectors of the economy compete for the same resources and may lay claim to the possibility that a shift in expenditures away from the healthcare industry toward other sectors may actually do more to improve the overall health of a nation. For example, greater access to education is linked to better health. Relatively inexpensive public health interventions decrease the spread of communicable disease and improve the health of those with limited resources. Personal choice and lifestyle modifications significantly decrease the incidence of chronic disease. On a global level, the need to care for people with HIV/AIDS and to decrease its incidence remains a serious challenge.

PHYSICAL ENVIRONMENT

Structural Design and Renovation

The physical environment in which healthcare services are provided is important to the healing process. Patients and their families voice approval or disapproval of their surroundings and relate the comfort of the care setting to the overall quality of care provided. Healthcare design has become its own subspecialty within the healthcare industry.

Design specialists are working on the creation of safe, attractive environments, most notably in the area of LTC and Alzheimer's disease and dementia care facilities. Wellness communities and models such as Planetree, which has "healing and nurturing mind, body and spirit" as part of its mission (Planetree, 2009), are having an influence on the more mainstream sector of the healthcare design business. The purposeful use of color, texture, light, and sound contribute to patients' sense of well-being as well as that of the staff. Settings designed with the functions of the staff in mind contribute to employees' efficiency and to a decrease in their illnesses or injuries.

Participant Roles

The list of those involved in the design of the physical environment in which health care takes place is virtually endless. Frontline staff and managers as well as project managers, architects, design engineers, construction engineers, safety and regulatory experts, physicians and other clinicians, executive-level decision-makers, and financial analysts are called on to participate in some way in the design process.

It is important that those who participate in various aspects of the design process are clear about their roles. For most managers and frontline staff, the role is consultative, not decision-making. The input of frontline personnel is essential because they are most familiar with day-to-day workflow. On the other hand, the expertise of architects and design engineers is needed to create a functional space in compliance with the countless regulatory mandates in which the care will take place.

Occupancy Approval

Before patients can occupy any bed in a healthcare facility, approval for occupancy must be granted. Generally, occupancy approval is part of the licensing process and rests with the state government, although local surrogates (for example, a designated local fire chief) may participate in the preliminary and final review process.

Architectural Review

The regulatory requirements for healthcare institution construction or remodeling are among the most stringent in existence. Not only must the initial plan undergo scrutiny at numerous levels, but every change, even the smallest adjustment, must undergo review and be approved in advance of construction. Adjustments that occur after construction begins are similarly subject to close review and approval.

Safety and Code Requirements

Federal and state agencies govern the safety of the environments in which care is provided. The Occupational Safety and Health Administration is the predominant federal agency concerned with the codes that pertain to healthcare environments. Each state has a parallel agency that is customized to the particular needs of that state. For example, a state known to experience earthquakes is likely to have a stricter code of seismic safety than one in which earthquakes do not pose a threat.

Because of the purpose, clientele, and the potential risk for harm to clients in healthcare environments, healthcare safety codes are extremely rigorous. Organizations must have systems and processes in place to assure compliance with all code requirements and must test their systems on an ongoing basis.

Efficiency

Environmental design should contribute to the efficiency of practice in a given unit. On one hand, the unit should be designed to accommodate the needs of the patients who will be housed and the staff who will practice there. On the other hand, given the dynamic nature of health care, a unit designed exclusively with today's patient or staff population in mind may be obsolete before the doors open.

Still, a few principles are relatively universal and constant over time:

- Staff should be able to see as many patients as possible from their assigned workstation.
- Patients should be provided with privacy and quiet; family needs should be considered.
- Sufficient storage space can ensure that the appearance of the unit is not cluttered.
- Workstations should meet stringent ergonomic standards, including proper lighting.
- The work unit should conserve energy for the staff (e.g., if long halls are necessary because of design constraints, workstations should be decentralized).

Effects on Clients and Staff

Florence Nightingale identified the positive effects of a pleasing environment on health, healing, and well-being. Ancient practitioners, too, identified the importance of creating pleasant surroundings as part of the art of healing.

Research into the design and furnishing of LTC facilities is currently a robust field. Whenever possible, clients or potential clients are involved in the design process. The intentional use of color, artwork, lighting, and sound create an atmosphere that can contribute to the well-being of staff and patients.

Case Study

A CNO wants OB nurses to begin doing c-sections in OB rather than having them done in the operating room. This will be a major change in practice. How can the CNO begin the change process for this major change initiative?

REFERENCES

Agency for Healthcare Research and Quality. (2009). *Home page*. Retrieved from http://www.ahrq.gov/

American Nurses Association. (2000). *Scope and standards of practice for nursing professional development.* Washington, DC: American Nurses Publishing.

American Nurses Association. (2003). *Nursing's social policy statement* (2nd ed.). Washington, DC: American Nurses Publishing.

American Nurses Association. (2004). *Scope and standards for nurse administrators* (2nd ed.). Washington, DC: American Nurses Publishing.

American Nurses Association. (2008). *Nursing informatics: Scope and standards of practice.* Silver Spring, MD: American Nurses Publishing.

Bateman, T., & Snell, S. (2002). *Management: Competing in the new era* (5th ed.). Boston: McGraw-Hill/Irwin.

Benner, P. (2001). *From novice to expert: Excellence and power in clinical nursing practice.* (Commemorative ed.). Menlo Park, CA: Addison-Wesley.

Blanchard, K. H., & Johnson, S. (1982). *The one-minute manager.* New York: William Morrow.

Burns, N., & Grove, S. (2002). *Understanding nursing research* (3rd ed.). Philadelphia: W. B. Saunders.

Campbell, J. P., Maxey, V. A., & Watson, W. A. (1995). Hawthorne effect: Implications for prehospital research. *Annuals of Emergency Medicine, 26,* 590–594.

Carter, J. H. (2008). *Electronic health records: A guide for clinicians and administrators* (2nd ed.). Philadelphia: American College of Physicians.

Covey, S. (1989). *Seven habits of highly effective people.* New York: Free Press.

Deming, W. E. (2000). *Out of the crisis.* Cambridge: Massachusetts Institute of Technology Press.

Dye, C. (2000). *Leadership in health care: Values at the top.* Chicago: Health Administration Press.

Edwards, D. F. (1999). The Synergy Model: Linking patient needs to nurse competencies. *Critical Care Nurse, 19*(1), 88–90.

Fawcett, J. (2005). *Contemporary nursing knowledge: Analysis and evaluation of nursing theories.* Philadelphia: F. A. Davis.

Finkelman, A. W. (2006). *Leadership and management in nursing.* Upper Saddle River, NJ: Pearson/Prentice Hall.

Gebbie, K. (2009). 20th century reports on nursing and nursing education: What difference did they make? *Nursing Outlook, 57*(2), 84–92.

Harris, M. (1998). *Basic statistics for behavioral science research* (2nd ed.). Boston: Allyn & Bacon.

Heidi, S., Spence-Laschinge, H. K., & Finegan, J. (2008). Nursing professional practice environments: Setting the stage for constructive conflict resolution and work effectiveness. *Journal of Nursing Administration, 38*(5), 250–257.

Henry J. Kaiser Family Foundation. (2008). *Employee health benefits: 2008 annual survey.* Menlo Park, CA: Author.

Hood, L. J. (2009). *Leddy & Pepper's conceptual bases of professional nursing* (7th ed.). Philadelphia: Lippincott Williams & Wilkins.

Huber, D. (2006). *Leadership and nursing care management* (3rd ed.). Philadelphia: Saunders/Elsevier.

The Joint Commission. (n.d.). Citation standards. In The Joint Commission, *Joint Commission on Hospital Accreditation Manual.* Oak Brook, IL: Author.

Keehan, S., Sisko, A., Truffer, C., Smith, S., Cowan, C., Poisal, J., ... the National Health Expenditure Accounts Projections Team. (2008.). Health spending projections through 2017: The baby-boom generation is coming to Medicare. *Health Affairs Web Exclusive, 27*(2), W145–W155. Available at http://content.healthaffairs.org/cgi/content/abstract/27/2/w145

Kolcaba, K. (2002). *Comfort theory and practice: A vision for holistic health care and research.* New York: Springer.

Kouzes, J., & Posner, B. (1996). Seven lessons for leading the voyage to the future. In F. Hesselbein, M. Goldsmith, & R. Beckhard (Eds.), *The leader of the future* (pp. 99–110). San Francisco: Jossey-Bass.

Lim, J. S., & O'Connor, M. (1995). Judgemental adjustment of initial forecasts: Its effectiveness and biases. *Journal of Behavioral Decision Making, 8*, 149–168.

Longest, B., Rakich, J., & Darr, K. (2000). *Managing health services organizations and systems* (4th ed.). Baltimore, MD: Health Professions Press.

Marquis, B., & Huston, C. (2009). *Leadership roles and management functions in nursing: Theory and application.* Philadelphia: Lippincott Williams & Wilkins.

Marriner-Tomey, A., & Alligood, M. (2002). *Nursing theorists and their work* (5th ed.). St. Louis, MO: Mosby.

Mayer, P., & Salovey, J. D. (1990). Emotional intelligence. *Imagination, Cognition, and Personality, 9*, 185–211.

Morrison, I. (2002). *Health care in the new millennium: Vision, values, and leadership.* San Francisco: Jossey-Bass.

Munhall, P. (2001). *Nursing research: A qualitative perspective* (3rd ed.). Boston: Jones & Bartlett.

National Institute of Standards and Technology. (2002). *Malcolm Baldrige National Quality Award—2002 Award Recipient, Health Care Category: SSM Health Care* [Press Release]. Gaithersburg, MD: Author. Retrieved from http://www.nist.gov/public_affairs/releases/ssmhealth.htm

Peplau, H. (1991). *Interpersonal relations in nursing: A conceptual frame of reference for psychodynamic nursing.* New York: Springer.

Planetree. (2009). *About Planetree.* Retrieved from http://www.planetree.org/about.html

Porter-O'Grady, T., & Malloch, K. (Eds.). *Innovation leadership: Creating the landscape of healthcare.* Sudbury, MA: Jones & Bartlett.

Potter, P., & Perry, A. (2001). *Fundamentals of nursing* (5th ed.). St. Louis, MO: Mosby.

Phillips, J. (1992). *How to think about statistics* (rev. ed.). New York: Freeman.

Schermerhorn, J., Hunt, J., & Osborn, R. (1995). *Scope and standards for nursing administration.* Washington, DC: American Nurses Publishing.

Schermerhorn, J., Hunt, J., & Osborn, R. (2002, December 2). *Seton nurses earn national nursing honor.* Retrieved from http://www.seton.net/about_seton/awards_certifications/

Schermerhorn, J. R., Hunt, J., & Osborn, R. N. (2008). *Organizational behavior* (10th ed.). Hoboken, NJ: John Wiley & Sons.

Senge, P. (1990). *The fifth discipline: The art and practice of the learning organization.* New York: Doubleday.

Seton Healthcare Network. (2009). *Nursing at Seton.* Retrieved from http://www.seton.net/employment/nursing/nursing_at_seton/

Sullivan, E., & Decker, P. (2000). *Effective leadership and management in nursing* (5th ed.). Upper Saddle River, NJ: Prentice Hall.

Swansburg, R., & Swansburg, R. J. (2002). *Introduction to management and leadership for nurse managers* (3rd ed.). Boston: Jones & Bartlett.

Tappen, R. (2001). *Essentials of nursing leadership and management.* Philadelphia: F. A. Davis.

Thomas, S., & O'Kane, M. (2012). Value-based purchasing. *American Journal of Managed Care, 18*(11), 1–2.

Patient Protection and Affordable Care Act, Pub. L. No. 111-148, §2702, 124 Stat. 119, 318-319. (2010). Retrieved from http://dpc.senate.gov/healthreformbill/healthbill52.pdf

Tomey, A. M., & Alligood, M. R. (2006). *Nursing theorists and their work.* St. Louis, MO: Mosby.

Umiker, W. (1994). *Management skills for the new health care supervisor* (2nd ed.). Gaithersburg, MD: Aspen.

Walton, M., & Deming, E. (1988). *Deming management method.* New York: Perigee.

CHAPTER 3

HEALTHCARE ENVIRONMENT: INNOVATION, TECHNOLOGY, AND LEGAL ISSUES IN NURSING

INNOVATION AND HEALTHCARE TECHNOLOGY

Leading in the 21st century requires innovation and adaptation to the environment. Innovation may involve a simple change or a radical redesign of the system, but using something different seems to be the answer (Warner & Burton, 2009). To prepare competent practitioners, versed in the practice environment today, innovation is necessary in nursing practice and nursing education.

Innovation is defined as creativity that is characterized by originality and expressiveness, according to the American Heritage Dictionary of the English Language (2009). Innovation is that essential component of nursing practice that permits response and adaptation to the many variables presented in the practice environment. Innovation and creativity support dynamic nursing practice; creativity is enhanced with intrinsic motivation, a nurturing environment, an ability to function independently, and a willingness to take risks (Fasnacht, 2003).

A leader can enhance creativity by building an environment of trust and interpersonal relationships, along with promoting a willingness to listen and spirit of cooperation. In addition, according to Longo (2013), key strategies to enhancing creativity include providing time for educational offerings, providing time for creative work, and encouraging calculated risk-taking and acceptance of personal responsibility.

Risk-Taking and Changing the Healthcare Environment

Leaders as coaches can support risk-taking by welcoming calculated risks into the work environment and encouraging positive risk-taking. The benefits of taking the risk for employees provides practice and participation in decision-making, increases confidence, increases a sense of control, decreases anxieties and fears, and can increase motivation.

Taking risk is engaging in behaviors that have potential to be harmful or dangerous, yet at the same time provide opportunity for some kind of outcome that can be perceived as positive (Tull, 2009). *Risk* in general can be defined as the "effect of uncertainty on objectives." Uncertainties include events (which may or may not happen) and uncertainties caused by ambiguity or a lack of information. It also includes both negative and positive effects on objectives (ISO 31000, 2009).

As Mark Twain said, "Twenty years from now you will be more disappointed by the things you didn't do than by the ones you did. So throw off the bowlines, sail away from the safe harbor, catch the trade winds in your sails. Explore. Dream. Discover" (Twain, n.d.).

Technology as an Innovation That Affects Practice

Technology to compute information has roughly doubled every 14 months between 1986 and 2007. Information technology as an integral part of life encompasses communication, documentation, and consumerism. Today the terms "information technology" and "informatics" are interchangeable. The primary goal of information technology is simply information management.

Continued developments in informatics support advances in clinical care, administration management, research, and education.

The goal of technology is to have the right information always available at the right time. Data management supports informed decision-making. Information systems provide leaders and managers with day-to-day information on patient flow and acuity, resource use, staffing levels, and costs and budgetary balance. There continue to be advances in moving healthcare information technology forward in the form of national forces, nursing forces, patient safety, and cost.

The national forces at work began with the creation of the President's Information Technology Advisory Committee in 2005, which became the Office of Science and Technology in 2012. The timeline for electronic health records (EHRs) began with a call for their use in 2004. Federal legislation under President George W. Bush required that all medical health records be electronic by 2014, and provided initial subsidies to make this happen. This was the same timeline for establishment of National Coordinator for Health Information Technology (NCHIT), a part of which was the creation of the 2008–2012 Strategic Plan with two goals addressing healthcare delivery: patient-focused health care and population health.

The goal of patient-focused health care is to provide higher quality, cost-effective care using electronic information exchange among healthcare providers, patients, and their designees. The strategic plan to reach this goal requires facilitating electronic exchange of health information while preserving privacy and security, increasing interoperable exchange of information, promoting nationwide adoption of EHRs and personal health records, and establishing collaborative governance guiding health information technology infrastructure.

The goal of population health allows for access and use of electronic health information to support public health, biomedical research, quality improvement, and emergency preparedness. The strategic plan to reach this goal requires advancing privacy and security policies, principles, procedures, and protections for information access in population health. Reaching the goal of population health also will require enabling an exchange of health information to support population-oriented uses, promoting nationwide adoption of technologies to improve population and individual health, and establishing coordinated organizational processes supporting information use for population health.

Nursing Forces at Work

Nursing continues to help drive healthcare information technology along a timeline:

- 1993: National Center for Nursing Research
    - Building clinical databases
    - Methods to evaluate nursing information systems
- 1997: National Agenda for Education & Practice
    - Educate nurses in core informatics content
- American Association of College of Nursing (2006-2008-2011)
    - Core competencies in healthcare technologies

Healthcare information technology contributes to evidence-based care through a standardization of terminologies and structure in documentation. In addition, the use of digital information, the standards allowing for data exchange between heterogenous entities, the ability to capture data relevant to actual care provided, and competency among practitioners to use data will all contribute to evidence-based care (Bakken, 2001).

The Institute of Medicine (IOM) Reports (2001–2003) support the use of healthcare information technology to improve practices and promote patient safety. Informatics is a core competency for all healthcare professionals and is seen as an important force in improving health care. Areas of focus for the IOM center on:

- National information infrastructure
- Computerized clinical data
- Clinical decision support
- Use of the Internet
- Integration of evidence-based practice.

The American Nurses Association also has promoted the use of healthcare information technology beginning with the 1994's *Standards of Practice for Nursing Informatics* and *Scope of Practice for Nursing Informatics.* In addition, the Committees for Nursing Practice Information Infrastructure and National Information and Data Set Evaluation Center are in place to support nursing practice with technology.

PATIENT SAFETY AS A DRIVING FORCE FOR HEALTHCARE INFORMATION TECHNOLOGY

Many patient safety databases use aggregated data to identify safety issues. Examples include the vaccine adverse event reporting system through the Centers for Disease Control and Prevention (CDC), the U.S. Food & Drug Administration, the National Nosocomial Infection Surveillance System through the CDC, and the Quality and Safety Initiative by Robert Wood Johnson Foundation (2010), which is based on IOM's five core competencies (patient-centered care, teamwork and collaboration, evidence-based practice, quality improvement, and informatics). Other processes that support safe practice and quality patient outcomes include using a bar coding system for medication administration and computerized provider order entry systems.

The Leapfrog Group (2000) was formed in response to high costs of health care without the ability to assess quality or compare healthcare providers, and consisted of large American corporations. Their 2009 mission was to improve safety, quality, and affordability of health care. They also work toward encouraging availability of information to consumers to facilitate informed healthcare decisions and using incentives and rewards to promote high-value health care. They collect voluntary data from healthcare organizations that they publish for consumer use on their website (Leapfrog Group 2009).

Increasing the Use of Healthcare Information Technology

Marketplace forces are driving increased use of healthcare information technology. Organizations are responding to the forces of competition, the need for economic survival in a competitive marketplace, the drive for professional accountability for the costs of diagnostic and therapeutic interventions and choices, and patient outcomes and satisfaction.

Meaningful Use for Healthcare Information Technology

Generally stated goals for the increased use of healthcare information technology include improving quality, safety, and efficiency. Technology is being used to engage patients and families in the process of healthcare delivery. Improving care coordination across the continuum of care helps to improve the overall health of the public and population at large. Meaningful use for healthcare technology also helps to ensure privacy and security for personal health information.

Requirements for Healthcare Information Technology

Today's requirements for effective healthcare technology can be condensed into an information technology system that can track and quantify the costs of care, the process of care, and the outcomes of care. There is also a need for information technology that can document the care being delivered in a fast, efficient, and consistent manner.

Investing in Nursing Informatics

Best practices include promoting the use of health information technology systems that improve documentation and reduce time spent on documentation. The best practice systems also provide patient data for quality improvement and provide patient data for research.

Supporting Practice

Four major domains of data in healthcare information technology support the delivery of care for the client, the provider, the leader, and research (Huber, 2010). Client care is supported through the client's medical record, including the evaluation process, the gathering of all clinical data, documentation of client outcomes, and achieved care outcomes. In addition, it is necessary to gauge client satisfaction and to assess and document the costs and access to care.

Healthcare information technology supports practice and the provider through personnel records and links to client records and national databases. General information that can be gathered includes professional data, caregiver outcomes, job enrichment opportunities, and job/work satisfaction. Information technology also provides an opportunity to gather information on physician satisfaction and job stress and/or intent to leave. There are opportunities to provide decision-maker variables and support for general care delivery through access to standards and databases.

Nurse leaders rely on administrative databases for issues related to management and resource oversight. Efficient practice is supported through access to databases containing real-time information in areas such as costs, productivity, turnover, and income. A global view of the organization includes databases that contain overall systems outcomes.

Healthcare information technology supports the evidence-based practice environment through existing and newly gathered data and relational databases. In general, the technology supports knowledge base development, practice-based evidence, and evidence-based practice. Research databases provide a clinical data repository, information, the ability to warehouse information, and an accessible data repository.

The Role of Nursing Informatics

Nursing informatics as a practice specialty is having a major impact on the way care is planned and delivered in the current healthcare environment. Nursing informatics refers to that component of informatics designed for and relevant to nurses and includes information management, knowledge from sciences other than nursing, and the importance of informatics within all areas of nursing practice.

The Specialty of Nursing Informatics

In a technologic world where information turns over rapidly, nursing informatics provides and facilitates nursing education in informatics and technology, and allows nurses to analyze, design, and implement information and communication systems. In addition, nursing informatics specialists, commonly referred to as *informaticists*, conduct and participate in effectiveness research to advance nursing epistemology.

Leadership Competencies in Healthcare Information Technology

Nurse leaders need a working knowledge of healthcare information management and technology, with a foundation in basic software skills (spreadsheets, word processing, email, social media, Internet use, and database management). Correctly used, technology supports financial management, process improvement, and quality improvement. Additionally, healthcare information technology supports general business intelligence and benchmarking for assessment and comparison of performance, while clinical information systems support the care delivery process.

Today's Healthcare and Information Technology

Documentation is an integral part of providing healthcare services today. Looking at the need for documentation for patient care and regulatory and accrediting bodies, a function of technology is to provide modification rather than redundancy of information and uniform rather than individualized care processes. Technology supports parallel rather than serial processing of patients through a transparency of technology. Technology and computers work their magic behind the scenes, where the user should perceive only the results and not the process unless so desired.

Technology and Documentation

Healthcare information technology provides for standardized language and terminology that improves quality outcomes and decreases medical errors. Documentation pathways link assessments, interventions, and outcomes for all users to provide the right information at the right time. Technology provides links to literature and nursing research to promote an evidence-based practice environment. Technology is changing the paradigm of documentation and promoting culture shifts, with increasing use of the electronic health record.

The American Nurses Association and Documentation Standardization Efforts

The American Nurses Association (ANA) has been actively involved in promoting standard documentation for healthcare records and nursing practice, beginning with the USA Nursing Minimum Data Sets (NMDS). The NMDS supports nursing care and patient demographics in nursing education, health information system designs, and clinical research. For leaders, the ANA has developed the Nursing Management Minimum Data Set (NMMDS), which provides data on the environment, nursing care, and financial resources and is used to obtain information to manage the environment and provide comparable data for benchmarking.

Management Information Systems

Management information systems (MISs), essential to the business of health care, represent an almost staggering investment of resources to ensure that the systems needed to conduct business, document clinical care, capture trends, and meet the demands of regulatory bodies and purchasers are in place. The rapidity with which technology is changing means not only an initial investment, but also ongoing capital and operational expenditures.

Organizations related to healthcare MISs have come into existence in recent years, as have careers in this area. Medical records administrators and clinical librarians are but two of the careers that have changed dramatically with the advent of MIS. Indeed, these job titles themselves are nearly obsolete. It is not uncommon to see a chief information officer (CIO) integrated into the executive level of the organizational chart of healthcare organizations.

The acronyms *WAN* (wide area network) and *LAN* (local area network) are common terms to the majority of administrators and clinicians alike. Now an entire vocabulary of technology terms sits alongside the medical lexicon.

Local area network refers to several personal computers linked together through a server. The concept is somewhat akin to an office that has several phone lines, each connected to the others, although able to be used independently.

Wide area networks are made up of LANs, and the system can be enlarged exponentially. Connections are affected by specialized networking software and are transparent to the user.

Nursing has its own association, the American Nursing Informatics Association, whose members are involved with or interested in the field of nursing informatics. The ANA describes *nursing informatics* as a scientific discipline that is broader in scope of practice and incorporates disciplines other than nursing, such as computer science and information science.

Electronic data transfer fosters the integration of care across the continuum. However, the promise of the fully functional computerized medical record is yet to be realized. As those who practice in the field of informatics have learned, the complexity of health care is such that the anticipated migration from paper to "bits and bytes" has yet to occur on a large scale.

Nonetheless, the *electronic health record* will eventually become a near-universal reality. An understanding of semantics related to the computerization of medical and health records is useful. The *automated medical record (AMR)* is considered a "first-level" product that brings together information from other sources. The AMR is delivered electronically to an end-user for her or his use in caring for the patient. However, the end-user cannot immediately enter data (respond to) what she or he has received (i.e., the AMR is not interactive).

The next level is termed the *computerized medical record system,* in which paper-based products now become available electronically through scanning. The *electronic medical record* is the third-level product; it provides capability for electronic data entry, electronic signature, data integrity, and audit tools. The *electronic patient record* is the fourth-level product; it brings together information about the patient from more than one organization, thus supporting the argument for a universally agreed-on "e-language" and code. Finally, the *electronic health record* is the fifth-level product, including information about the person's well-being from multiple sources, not only about her or his medical problem (Carter, 2008).

The Internet

The World Wide Web represents a phenomenon without parallel. The instantaneous availability of information and the ability to connect with the person next door or colleagues half a world away does indeed make planet Earth seem a bit smaller.

The Internet is changing the way medicine—and by extension, nursing—is practiced. Patients are engaged in self-care as never before. They approach their providers with the latest articles about illness, medications, treatments, and research in hand. Expectations have changed; relationships have been altered. While the concepts of *patient as partner* or *patient as leader of her or his health team* are not yet universally embraced, they are clearly on the horizon.

Telehealth is no longer in the realm of science fiction. The Office of the National Coordinator of Healthcare Technology now exists as a division within the Health Resources and Services Administration, itself a division of the U.S. Department of Health and Human Services (http://healthit.hhs.gov/portal/server.pt).

In telehealth, nurses use laptops and small video cameras to videotape the patient in her or his residence in real time. The recording can be transmitted immediately to other health-care providers so that assessment and needed intervention can occur in the moment. The transmission is not constrained by time or distance; thus, patients in remote locations can enjoy the same level of consultation as those who live adjacent to medical centers. Radiologists read digitized images from a location far removed from the diagnostic imaging department. Laboratory data are transmitted via secure servers from location to location.

Telehealth provides to real-time access to healthcare services. The patient and provider interact at the same time with the ability to store and forward communication to additional healthcare providers, if necessary. Telehealth facilitates electronic capture of diagnostics for specialist interpretation.

An extension of telehealth is *telehomecare*. Recognizing the need to provide access to services to clients in need, telehomecare is the ability to monitor and deliver care at home through a variety of services. Examples of telehomecare services include portable monitoring devices, automatic pill dispensers/reminders, and biometric garments.

Other examples of technology supporting the care environment include e-intensive care units for remote monitoring of critical care patients and teletrauma that is used in rural hospitals for second opinions and advice from trauma care experts. The goal in using the technology is to enhance patient care and provide access to healthcare services in rural areas of the country.

Telenursing

A new and developing specialty is *telenursing*. Telenursing is used in various settings, including colleges, hospitals, and healthcare insurers' patient outreach programs. The practice of telenursing creates more collaborative and autonomous roles for nurses and also contributes to cost-containment efforts.

Challenges to Telehealth/Telenursing

As new and emerging forms of care delivery develop, issues and challenges arise. Reimbursement and medico-legal issues, along with technical issues, are common challenges. There are opportunities for research as technology facilitates new forms of practice and outreach to determine the outcomes and effectiveness of new care delivery systems.

There are few barriers in the virtual world save for the electronic security "firewalls" purposely incorporated into information systems. Many organizations take advantage of the firewall concept to create intranet systems that allow communication only within defined boundaries.

As with any seemingly wondrous invention, the Internet also brings with it a cautionary tale. The accuracy and source of information must be carefully scrutinized. It is incumbent on healthcare professionals to assist patients and families in distinguishing information that is of high quality from that which is questionable or even harmful. Vigilance also is called for with regard to "hackers" who break into systems, sometimes with the intent to harm, at other times simply for the thrill of proving they can "scale the wall."

Technology as an Innovation

Innovation is nursing practice that permits response and adaptation to the many variables presented in the practice environment. Healthcare information technology is at the foundation of effective current practice, promoting effective management of resources for nurse leaders who are highly dependent on up-to-date and efficient use of information that requires integration of patient, staff, and economic variables.

Nursing is the largest and most labor-intensive component of hospital costs, using on average 50% of operating budgets. Nurses are also the most constant presence at point of care. Technology has been shown to promote patient safety, quality efforts, access to care, and cost containment. Nurse leaders are in a key position to be actively involved in all healthcare information technology activities to evaluate products and systems, lobby for the purchase of products and systems, and utilize all technology available to support care delivery in today's healthcare organizations.

Consumers and Electronic Health Records

As information technology changes nursing practice and health care, consumers will have to become a part of this paradigm shift in delivery practices. Technology sets the stage for consumers to begin taking more responsibility for their health care. Provider–patient relationships are changing as consumers become more informed, seek information on the Internet, and begin to maintain personal health records.

The personal health record provides individuals an ability to communicate with their authorized providers and maintain and manage their own personal health information. Three main formats currently exist: software applications for computer or flash drive, web-based services to store information remotely, and hybrids. The benefit of the personal health record is its ability to promote collaborative care and facilitate personal management of disease treatment. There are challenges to the personal health record that generally involve the issues of data security, data standards, and data presentation. There are also concerns related to costs, provider reluctance, and maintaining unique patient identifiers.

As with all new technologies, the challenges to personal health records are ones that will continue to be addressed as patients and providers increase in user numbers. Personal health records as a technology will support the continuum of care by providing the right information at the right time.

Healthcare information technology in general reaches beyond the walls of healthcare organizations and intensive care environments across the continuum of care to palliative care. Technology requires ongoing training on medical devices and ultimately managing medical technology in a patient-safe way.

LEGAL ISSUES IN PROFESSIONAL PRACTICE AND INSTITUTIONAL LIABILITIES

Law That Affects Organizations and Practice

Two areas of the law that most involve healthcare leaders and managers are employment law and malpractice. The major employment laws include the Family Medical Leave Act (FMLA), Civil Rights Act of 1964, the Age Discrimination in Employment Act of 1967, and Occupational Health and Safety Act (OSHA). The general liabilities related to these laws include violation of the FMLA, discrimination, retaliation, wrongful termination, wage and hour violations, and violations of OSHA. Strategies to decrease employment law liabilities include documentation of all issues and employee encounters; reporting up the chain of command; unilaterally enforcing policies, procedures, and laws; and consulting legal council. Laws and regulatory issues are covered in depth in Chapter 6.

Malpractice issues for nurse leaders include personal negligence in clinical practice; liability for delegation and supervision; and staffing issues such as adequate numbers of staff with increased patient acuity and limited resources, floating staff from one unit to another, and the use of temporary or agency staff to augment staffing. Nurse leaders are charged with a duty to orient, educate, and evaluate; failure to attend to these issues can result in malpractice claims. Nurse leaders also are charged with strict product liability for the actions of staff. Lastly, negligent hiring may be an area of malpractice if staff is hired without the appropriate license and credential verification.

Corporations have a duty and responsibility to their patients and staff. The duties implied include maintaining a safe facility and safe equipment; providing competent, qualified, trained, and licensed individuals to provide care; providing proper orientation and supervision of the staff; and maintaining appropriate policies, procedures, and bylaws. Additional responsibilities and liabilities include *respondeat superior* (vicarious liability); ostensible authority; corporate negligence; Emergency Medical Treatment and Active Labor Act (EMTALA) claims; and mandatory reporting at the federal and state level for issues of neglect, child abuse, and elder abuse.

Tort Law and Medical Malpractice

Tort law includes negligence and professional negligence. A *tort* is a civil wrong that allows the injured individual to seek damages. Damages (compensation) are paid to the injured by the individual who caused the harm. Tort law is civil law and protects others from unreasonable and foreseeable risks of harm. A tort is a civil wrong other than breach of conduct and civil law provides a remedy for injured person to seek damages.

Types of torts include both negligence and professional negligence. *Negligence* is conduct falling below legal standards that protect members of society from harm. Professional negligence is conduct of professionals that falls below a professional standard of due care. Torts include assault and battery, libel and slander, and wanton and willful conduct.

Professional negligence varies in definition from state to state. Professional negligence is generally described as a failure to apply a professional standard of care. Medical malpractice is professional negligence. In professional negligence, a nurse's conduct is compared to what a reasonable nurse would do in the same situation/circumstance.

The terms *negligence* and *malpractice* are sometimes confused with one another or assumed to be synonymous. This is not the case. *Negligence* is

- The failure to do what a reasonably careful and prudent person would do under the same or like circumstances *(omission)* or
- The doing of something that a reasonably careful and prudent person would not do under the same or like circumstances *(commission).*

Briefly, negligence is the failure to exercise reasonable or ordinary care.

Malpractice goes beyond negligence. Four elements must be present for malpractice to occur:

- *Duty:* How would a reasonable and prudent provider behave under the same circumstances?
- *Breach of duty:* Did the provider breach the standard of care in this particular situation?
- *Causation:* Was the unreasonable, careless, or inappropriate behavior on the part of the provider the proximate cause of the injury or insult?
- *Injury:* Did injury to the patient/client occur?

If any one of these elements cannot be proved "beyond a reasonable doubt," then a malpractice claim may be dismissed.

Professional negligence claims against nurses are based almost exclusively on personal injury. These claims also have resulted from various types of negligent conduct. Current negligence claims have involved product liability and, most recently, complementary/alternative healthcare options suggested by nurses to patients for personal use.

Defenses against allegations of professional negligence include untimely filing of the case (filing after the statute of limitations runs out) and an assumption of risk whereby the plaintiff knew "it" was dangerous, had facts about the danger, and chose to take on the danger. Another defense is immunity from suit such as the common "Good Samaritan act." Overall, the best strategies for prevention of malpractice include striving for continued best practices, and being professional, pleasant, and people-oriented.

A charge of negligence can arise from any action or failure to act that results in patient injury. Most often this occurs from an unintentional failure to adhere to a standard of clinical practice. The best defense is a good offense. Knowing the factors contributing to the increase in the number of malpractice cases against nurses helps to build a good defense, and in today's health care, the greatest number of cases are reported in acute care healthcare organizations, followed by long-term-care facilities (nursing homes, rehabilitation facilities, transitional care units).

Insurance

Two types of liability are of concern to those in the health professions: (1) personal liability and (2) corporate liability. *Personal liability* holds that individuals are responsible for their own actions. *Vicarious liability* is an extension of personal liability and holds that certain parties may not be negligent themselves, but their negligence is assumed because of association with the negligent individual. *Corporate liability* holds that an organization is responsible for its conduct.

Healthcare organizations are, by the nature of their business, heavily insured to protect against liability and, by extension, their employees also are insured. The doctrine of *respondeat superior* (let the master speak) allows the courts to hold employers responsible for the actions of the organization's employees when the employees are performing services for the organization. This concept sometimes gives nurses and other healthcare professionals a false sense of security in that they assume they cannot be sued individually in the case of actual or perceived wrongdoing. Indeed, patients may sue both the institution and the individual practitioner. Thus, nurses are advised to carry their own personal liability insurance.

Documentation

The need for precise, accurate documentation has been reinforced repeatedly in the field of nursing. "If it's not documented, it's not done" is an oft-repeated mantra within the profession. New challenges lie ahead as computerized documentation systems become more widespread without benefit of standardized rules, processes, and technical languages. Although such guidelines will come in time through various regulatory bodies, the initial products are being activated at the institutional level. At the present time, electronic documentation systems are no more consistent than their paper-and-pencil counterparts (Smith, Smith, Krugman, & Oman, 2005).

The Medical Record

Documentation takes place in the form of a patient's medical record. The medical record serves as a complete and accurate record of a patient's condition. The record also serves as a basis for evaluating healthcare operations resources by providing research data and helping to determine reimbursement by third-party payers.

The medical record is a legal document and admissible in a court of law and provides a summary of a patient's hospital stay with treatments and outcomes noted. The record is generally owned by the hospital, but the patient owns the information it contains. The record is confidential and should not be discussed with anyone not in direct care of the patient.

In general, the medical record should be documented accurately and in a timely fashion and should contain elements of assessments, plan of care, medical interventions, and evaluations of the treatments. The record can assist with a malpractice defense if completed appropriately, or can hinder a malpractice defense if documented poorly. Defense attorneys value accurate, clear, and concise documentation and consider the medical record to be the best defense in a malpractice suit.

Legal Impact of Medical Errors

The Institute of Medicine reports that medical error is the leading cause of death in the United States. As currently reported, more people die from medical errors than from breast cancer, HIV, or motor vehicle crashes. The Archives of Internal Medicine reports that medication errors occur nearly 1 out of every 5 doses. Factors in the healthcare environment, including cognitive lapses (e.g., lack of attention, interruptions, "slips"), a tendency to generalize, confirmation bias, and overconfidence, contribute to medical errors.

Factors Affecting the Practice Environment and Liability

Nurse leaders are faced with challenges in the healthcare environment due to financial constraint and constriction of the environment. Greater productivity and efficiency challenge access to healthcare services while the public demands equitable access and funded healthcare services. In addition, there are changes in healthcare reimbursement based on government policy.

The litigious environment of health care is affected by the fact that the public and citizens know their rights relating to health care. They are more knowledgeable about health matters and are aware of government intervention and policies regarding patient involvement in care. Patients have the right to participate in decision-making matters relating to their health supported by law, and no longer accept the old paternalistic paradigm of healthcare delivery.

Another factor to consider in the review of legal issues is as simple as the aging population. People are living longer and, as a result, there are increasing numbers of older Americans with multiple healthcare needs and increasing numbers of aging Americans requiring complex care.

The last factor contributing to a complex legal environment for the delivery of health care is a shift in the practice setting from hospitals to primary care clinics, directed by government and reimbursement factors and the continual practice of transferring patients between acute and chronic care settings, and then back home as care needs change.

Nurse Leaders at the Forefront of Culture Change

Changing the culture paradigm is a responsibility of a nurse leader in today's healthcare environment. A strategy for changing the culture includes facilitating a move to assess events beyond blame, because errors do and will always occur. Other responsibilities relating to events include the duty to:

- Prevent events/errors when possible
- Report events
- Remedy injuries related to events
- Promote a culture of safety.

Other strategies to change the culture include promoting identification of safety issues as opportunities for performance improvement, ensuring a non-punitive environment for event reporting, reinforcing communication within the healthcare team and with patients and families, and encouraging patients to participate in their care.

Nurses must recognize the fact that today's healthcare environment contributes to the rise in malpractice claims against nurses. Increased autonomy and responsibility of nurses bring about greater risk of error and liability. Effective risk control strategies begin with the personal responsibilities of maintaining competencies and nursing skills through continuing education efforts; ensuring accurate, objective, and thorough documentation in all records; and examining personal professional practice to understand the challenges and risks.

Keeping current with the most common personal and organizational allegations is a good place to begin, because nurse leaders can identify their own vulnerabilities in the practice environment and take appropriate action to protect their practice and license.

REFERENCES

American Nurses Association. (2004). *Scope and standards for nurse administrators* (2nd ed.). Washington, DC: American Nurses Publishing.

American Nurses Association. (2006). *Scope and standards of nursing informatics practice.* Silver Spring, MD: Nursebooks.org.

American Nurses Association. (2008). *Nursing informatics: Scope and standards of practice.* Silver Spring, MD: American Nurses Publishing.

Bakken, S. (2001). An informatics infrastructure is essential for evidence-based practice. *Journal of the American Medical Informatics Association, 8*(3), 199–201.

Benner, P. (2001). *From novice to expert: Excellence and power in clinical nursing practice.* (commemorative ed.). Menlo Park, CA: Addison-Wesley.

Brandi, J. (2003). *Nine ways to engage staff and please the customer.* Retrieved from http://www.customerfocusconsult.com/articles/articles_template.asp?ID=47

Bobinski, M. A., Hall, M. A., & Orentlicher, D. (2007). *Health care law and ethics* (7th ed.). New York: Wolters Kluwer/Aspen

Carter, J. H. (2008). *Electronic health records: A guide for clinicians and administrators* (2nd ed.). Philadelphia: American College of Physicians.

Editors of The American Heritage® Dictionary of the English Language. (2009). *The American Heritage® Dictionary of the English Language* (4th ed.). Boston: Houghton Mifflin.

Fashnacht, P. H. (2003). Creativity: A refinement of the concept for nursing practice. *Journal of Advanced Nursing, 41*(2), 195–202.

Huber, D. (2010). *Leadership and nursing care management* (4th ed.). Philadelphia: Saunders/Elsevier.

Idea Champions. (2012). *50 awesome quotes on risk taking.* Retrieved from http://www.ideachampions.com/weblogs/archives/2011/03/security_is_mos.shtml

Ironside, P., & Valiga, T. M. (2007). How innovative are we? What is the nature of our innovation? *Nursing Education Perspectives, 28*(1), 51–53.

ISO Store: Standards Catalog. (2012). *ISO 31000:2009 Risk management: Principles and guidelines.* Retrieved from http://www.iso.org/iso/catalogue_detail.htm?csnumber=43170

Keehan, S., Sisko, A., Truffer, C., Smith, S., Cowan, C., Poisal, J., et al. (2008, February 26). Health spending projections through 2017: The Baby-Boom generation is coming to Medicare. *Health Affairs Web Exclusive,* W145–W155. Available at http://content.healthaffairs.org/cgi/content/abstract/27/2/w145

Leadershipnow.com. (2012). *Risk taking quotes.* Retrieved from http://www.leadershipnow.com/risktakingquotes.html

Leapfrog Group. (2009). *About Leapfrog.* Retrieved from http://www.leapfroggroup.org/about_leapfrog.

Longo, A. (2013). Change, complexity, and creativity. In L. Roussel (Ed.), *Management and leadership for nurse administrators* (6th ed., pp. 122–159). Burlington, MA: Jones & Bartlett Learning.

National Institutes of Health: Center for Information Technology. (n.d.). *Strategic plan 2008–2012.* Retrieved from http://cit.nih.gov/NR/rdonlyres/54A93894-A76C-4742-A559-421738E78557/0/CITStrategicPlan2008Final.pdf

Nigro, N. (n.d.). Coaches as risk takers: Coaching and mentoring. *Netplaces*. Retrieved from http://www.netplaces.com/coaching-mentoring/managing-diversity/coaches-as-risk-takers.htm

Porter-O'Grady, T., & Malloch, K. (Eds). (2009). *Innovation leadership: Creating the landscape of healthcare.* Sudbury, MA: Jones & Bartlett.

Planetree. (2009). *About Planetree.* Retrieved from http://www.planetree.org/about.html

Reising, D. L. & Allen, P. A. (2007, February). Protecting yourself from malpractice claims. *American Nurse Today*, 2(2), 39–44. Retrieved from http://www.americannursetoday.com/article.aspx?id=4186&fid=4172

Seton Healthcare Network. (2009). *Nursing at Seton.* Retrieved from http://www.seton.net/employment/nursing/nursing_at_seton/

Sewell, J., & Thede, L. (2013). *Informatics and nursing: opportunities and challenges* (4th ed.). Philadelphia:Wolters-Kluwer/Lippincott, Williams & Wilkins.

Sherfield, R.M. (n.d.) *Taking positive risks.* Retrieved from http://www.netplaces.com/self-esteem/expanding-your-comfort-zone/taking-positive-risks.htm

Smith, K., Smith, V., Krugman, M., & Oman, K. (2005). Evaluating the impact of computerized clinical documentation. *Computer Informatics Nursing, 23*(3), 132–138.

Tull, M. (2009). Impulsive behaviors: Managing impulsive behaviors. *About.com Guide.* Retrieved from http://ptsd.about.com/od/selfhelp/qt/impulsecope.htm

Twain, M. (n.d.). *Discovery.* Retrieved from http://www.twainquotes.com/Discovery.html

U. S. Department of Health and Human Services. (2012). *Update on the adoption of health information technology and related efforts to facilitate the electronic use and exchange of health information: A report to Congress.* Retrieved from http://healthit.hhs.gov/portal/server.pt/gateway/PTARGS_0_0_4383_1239_15610_43/http%3B/wci-pubcontent/publish/onc/public_communities/p_t/resources_and_public_affairs/reports/reports_portlet/files/january2012__update_on_hit_adoption_report_to_congress.pdf

Warner, J. R., & Burton, D. A. (2009). The policy and politics of emerging academic-service partnerships. *Journal of Professional Nursing, 25*(6), 329–334.

CHAPTER 4

HEALTHCARE ENVIRONMENT

High-quality healthcare organizations are driven by attention to their customers, excellent workmanship, empowered workforces, and innovation and change as a response to their environment. The forces that drive change in healthcare organizations also will drive change in society and life in the 21st century. Products and services must be needs-based, yet maintain a distinct identity to keep a company sustainable and in front of the competition. High-quality healthcare organizations recognize the factors that will allow them to be successful: team building, group dynamics, conflict resolution, negotiation, sources of power and empowerment, and other environmental issues.

TEAM BUILDING

"A team remains the most flexible and most powerful unit of performance, learning, and change in any organization" (Katzenbach & Smith, 2003, p. XIX). The abilities to express one's ideas clearly and decisively, to listen attentively and respectfully, and to invite a range of opinions are among the communication skills that help managers build team cohesiveness. Teams usually are developed reflecting the diversity and culture of the organization, and although the chief executive may be fundamental in the formation of high-performance teams, he or she is not always a team leader.

According to Katzenbach and Smith (2003), developing a team is the inclusion of "a small number of people with complementary skills who are committed to a common purpose, performance goals, and approach for which they hold themselves mutually accountable" (p. 275). A team develops around the task to be accomplished while taking into account the mix of personalities and competencies; the desired performance outcomes; and the processes of communication, involvement, performance orientation, and enabling leadership (Higgs, 2006).

Central to a team's success will be its members' work behaviors such as constructive listening and giving the benefit of the doubt to others (Katzenbach & Smith, 2003). Team members need to not only be mature and self-motivated, but also be aware of their social and cultural differences, appreciate each other's cultural diversity, and have a basic understanding for each other's value systems. Only through an active display of this understanding and open and nonjudgmental communication can a team develop its highest potential to meet group goals and complete its mission.

The team leader can facilitate this process by using good meeting skills and appropriate meeting behaviors. The task of reminding team members of their mission, goal, and tasks falls to the leader as well.

GROUP DYNAMICS

Social scientists have identified predictable stages of group development. The first stage is known as *forming*. Individuals come together and form a defined cluster. People are cautious in their communication with one another; they are still relative strangers and rely on a leader to define and direct their activities.

As the group proceeds through the maturation process, it arrives at the second stage known as *storming*. In this stage, members of the group compete for position, power, and status; informal leaders may emerge. The formal leader helps the group identify and work through conflict.

The third stage of group formation is called *norming*. Here the rules for working collaboratively are made explicit; structure, roles, and relationships are clarified. The leader's role is to advance relationship building.

As the group matures, it enters the *performing* stage; it is in this mode that the work of the group is done most effectively. The energy of the group is focused on achieving its goals in a collaborative atmosphere. The leader's role is to provide feedback on the work that the group is accomplishing, redirect group energy when necessary, and further cultivate interpersonal relationships.

Several experts have suggested that the group formation process, and thus, the productivity of the group, can be accelerated under the guidance of a skillful facilitator or in the face of actual or fabricated crisis.

CONFLICT AND CONFLICT RESOLUTION

Conflict occurs naturally in and among groups and individuals; it is inevitable and a condition essential to change. Conflict may be *intrapersonal* (within oneself), *interpersonal* (between the self and another person), *intragroup* (among members of a particular group), or *intergroup* (among members of two or more groups). Other types of conflict include *competitive* conflict and *disruptive or destructive* conflict. In both instances, the desired outcome is to overcome one's opponent (i.e., to "win").

Conflict management occupies a significant portion of a leader's work. Some suggest that at least one-quarter of the leader's time is spent in conflict management activities. The challenge for the leader is, of course, to help her or his subordinates reach a "win–win" outcome in which the parties to the conflict each believe they have come away from the encounter with a sense of resolution. Strategies include

- Focusing on goals, not personalities;
- Meeting the needs of both parties, equally if at all possible; and
- Building consensus.

Achieving a win–win outcome is much easier in the abstract than in the workplace setting. Nonetheless, it is a worthwhile goal.

Conflict is defined as a state of disharmony or clash. Managing conflict requires maintaining the level of conflict neither too high nor too low, with the ultimate goal being to stimulate growth and coping behavior without reaching the point where the conflict seems overwhelming. Common conflict resolution strategies include compromising, competing, cooperating, smoothing, avoiding, or collaborating (Marquis & Huston, 2009). *Confrontation* is a technique used to address specific issues, in part by developing a plan for employee behavior. That plan becomes the objective measure of change and needs to contain a follow-up to the initial meeting. If the behavior plan fails to resolve the conflict with the employee, the disciplinary process will more than likely be the next step.

NEGOTIATION

Negotiation can be thought of as a formal process; one example is the negotiations that take place at the time of contract deliberations between unions and management. Negotiation also can be thought of as a political process in that it is a "power play" among individuals who compete to "win" but generally compromise in the end. The key to successful negotiations include the principles of

- Separating the people from the problem;
- Focusing on interests, not positions;
- Inventing options for mutual gains; and
- Insisting on objective criteria.

Interest-based negotiation is a somewhat newer concept, the principles of which were outlined by Fisher, Ury, and Patton (1991) in *Getting to Yes: Negotiating Agreement Without Giving In*. Bizony (1999) has distilled the principles listed below from Fisher and colleagues' work on the Harvard Negotiation Project; their value has been convincingly promulgated through the years.

- Treat people as equals.
- Resolve issues on their merits.
- Define issues with a definition that is acceptable to all parties.
- Focus on interests, not on conclusions or positions.
- Develop options that may meet the interests of both parties.
- Apply objective standards to resolve conflicting interests.

Twelve points of negotiation can prepare leaders for successful negotiations.

- The greatest failure in negotiation is failing to negotiate.
- The most important person to know in negotiation is yourself.
- Everyone has power in negotiation.
- Single-issue bargaining leaves both parties unsatisfied.
- Urgency drives decisions.
- Agreement is the end; trade-offs are the means.
- The best results are obtained by keeping the other party on a need-to-know basis.
- The value of something is always in the eye of the beholder.
- Success in negotiation is directly related to the amount and kind of preparation preceding it.
- Being able to walk away or select an alternative to a negotiated agreement puts a negotiator in a very strong position.

- Two sides can always agree on something, even when they are far apart on major issues.
- Conflict is a part of meaningful negotiation.

Mediation as a method of dispute resolution uses a neutral third party who attempts to bring parties together to solve a conflict. The mediator's role is to fact find, make suggestions, and draft a solution that is agreeable to both parties (Epstein, 2003).

SOURCES OF POWER AND EMPOWERMENT

Power is the capacity to act and the energy to mobilize resources to create change. Whether power has a positive or a negative connotation depends on how it is used. Several types of power available to leaders have been identified.

- *Legitimate power* suggests that the leader has the right or authority to tell others what to do. The reciprocal nature of this power obligates employees to comply with legitimate orders.
- *Reward power* is exercised over others when the leader has the ability to compensate others in some way. Compensation need not be monetary.
- *Coercive power* indicates that the leader has the ability to punish those who are noncompliant.
- *Referent power* means that the leader has characteristics that appeal to others. People comply because they admire him or her or have a desire for approval.
- *Expert power* means that the leader has certain expertise or knowledge. People comply because they believe in or can otherwise gain from affiliation with the person with expert power.

All sources of power are potentially important, and the assumption is that the most powerful leaders are those who have high legitimate, reward, or coercive power. However, one should not underestimate the strength of referent and expertise power. These sources of power are more closely related to personal motivation and may, in the long run, make a greater and more lasting difference within a company or organization. Nor is it necessarily the leaders whose names are well known or who sit atop the organizational chart who exert the most power of this type.

In today's healthcare environment, where the span of control has been increased for most executives, it is important that all staff are empowered to make decisions, especially those decisions that affect positive patient care outcomes. Studies have previously documented that nurses like to function in autonomous roles. Such role functions must incorporate the concepts of power and empowerment.

ADAPTING TO CHANGE

Appreciative Inquiry

Appreciative inquiry is the process in which an organization asks questions of its members in seeking information that can be used to anticipate and identify areas of potential strengths. The four characteristics of appreciative inquiry include

- Appreciative,
- Applicable,
- Provocative, and
- Collaborative.

Appreciative inquiry is best described through the 4 Ds:

1. Discovering the best of what is,
2. Dreaming what might be,
3. Designing what should be, and
4. Creating a destiny of what will be.

Appreciative inquiry is to organizations what creative visualization is to individuals; both are positive approaches to foster change. Appreciative inquiry is considered to be a "soft business strategy" that can be used to create organizational visions, build cultures, and align groups to achieve organizational goals. Through imagination and thoughtful analysis, appreciative inquiry can contribute to measurable results for organizations.

Crisis Management

A *crisis* is anything that has the potential to significantly affect an organization. Organizations with crisis management plans are better able to work effectively with local responders, promptly attend to the needs of those affected, assist investigating bodies without jeopardizing the organization's legal position, provide for accurate and timely information, and minimize damage to the organization's reputation.

The four objectives of crisis management are

- Reducing tension during the incident;
- Demonstrating organizational commitment and expertise;
- Controlling the flow and accuracy of information; and
- Managing resources effectively.

Managing a crisis begins with the creation of a crisis management team and assessing potential crises before they occur. Managing a crisis also includes

- Developing crisis management team plans;
- Establishing guidelines for gathering information and beginning an internal investigation;
- Providing periodic crisis training evaluation; and
- Developing guidelines for crisis communication.

The key points for crisis management of any dimension include

- Having a flexible structure capable of responding to any crisis quickly, decisively, and in a coordinated manner;
- Preparing operational contingency plans;
- Creating and communicating a document retention policy (e.g., nothing is thrown away that might enhance an investigation or document the event);
- Developing training that includes addressing legal issues before they occur, developing investigational procedures, identifying necessary equipment and systems before a crisis, and developing good media relations skills;
- Preparing to communicate with a variety of constituents, including employees, the media, neighbors, investors, regulators, and lawmakers; and
- Preparing a business contingency plan to minimize disruption and damage.

Because crisis management is the manner in which organizations respond to unexpected events over which they have little or no control, and "uncontrollable" situations occur with relative frequency in health care, developing purposeful intervention strategies seems prudent. The "truthful disclosure" approach is one that healthcare organizations take to maintain public trust.

A classic example of a crisis management in healthcare products can be seen in the Johnson & Johnson's handling of the Tylenol® tampering crisis (Kaplan, 1998). In 1982, seven people in the Chicago area died after taking Extra-Strength Tylenol capsules that had been injected with cyanide. The containers had been tampered with after they left the manufacturing plant. Rather than claim that the company was not to blame, Johnson & Johnson immediately launched a public relations program to preserve the integrity of the product and the company.

Marketing experts believed that Tylenol would disappear from pharmacy shelves, never to be mentioned again except in negative terms. However, Johnson & Johnson's leaders put public safety first and worried about financial impact later. They alerted consumers throughout the nation to avoid the consumption of any Tylenol product until the extent of the tampering could be determined. They stopped production of all Tylenol products and recalled all Tylenol capsules from the market at a cost of more than $100 million. They offered to replace any Tylenol capsules people had already purchased with Tylenol tablets. They quickly began working with the Chicago Police Department, the Federal Bureau of Investigation, and the Federal Drug Administration. They put up $100,000 in reward money to help catch the perpetrator of the crime.

Not only did the company survive and thrive, Tylenol remains one of its biggest-selling and most profitable products. The forthright approach of the company reassured the community that its safety came first and that Johnson & Johnson cared enough to be publicly open and truthful about the crisis (Kaplan, 1998).

Crisis management by companies such as Qantas Airlines, Exxon-Mobil, and Boeing demonstrates the effectiveness of the four objectives of crisis management in responding to the crisis in an organized format, protecting an organization's reputation, communicating effectively through company channels to resolve the crisis, and normalizing operations following catastrophic events.

ENVIRONMENTAL FACTORS

Cultural Competence

Cultural competence can be defined as the ability to interact effectively with people of different cultures with a focus on personal awareness of one's own culture and attitude toward culture, and development of knowledge and skill across multiple cultures. Cultural competence is essential as a leadership strategy in today's healthcare environment. Our "shrinking" planet, globalization, and population movement bring people from different cultures throughout the world together in the workplace, and people may have widely divergent understandings of identity and society. Globalization has increased the need for awareness of cultural ideas and expectations other than our own in an environment where intermixing national, religious, and ethnic identities may lead to conflict.

The world's population is expected to double by 2050 (Kotlikoff & Burns, 2004). Industrialized nations are "graying," while 80% of the world's population growth is in developing nations. Challenges for the workplace include language and cultural differences, increasing incidence of chronic illness, generational issues, maximization of resource use, and ethical differences.

Strategies for success relating to cultural competence include

- Know your own culture, values, and biases.
- Listen and observe.
- Emphasize corporate values at all times.
- Be a teacher and a learner.
- Hold up your end of the bargain by displaying awareness of personal cultural practices.
- Give clear directions and provide resources.
- Delegate the responsibility for outcomes.
- Give the big picture.
- Consider the rules and procedures from all perspectives.

A leader's responsibility in cultural competence includes

- Managing personal expectations,
- Providing straightforward steps for decision-making,
- Being courageous and displaying correct behavior,
- Applying leadership and management skills according to values and attitudes, and
- Providing employees the opportunity to grow.

Because today's workforce consists of four generations (i.e., mature, baby boomers, generation x, millennials), a leader also must consider generational diversity as well as cultural diversity. There are challenges relating to work ethics, duty, and sacrifice for the job.

A leader's role in cultural and generational competence in today's healthcare organization includes

- Creating a culture that has a diversity-sensitive orientation;
- Building the blocks of culturally and linguistically competent healthcare delivery;
- Recruiting and retaining a diverse workforce; and
- Ensuring the success of a culturally competent organization.

Effective leaders are aware of and make use of cultural competence to maximize the benefits of diversity in their staff and patient population and minimize the costs in delivering healthcare services today. In nursing practice, nurse leaders should encourage members of other cultures to become nurses, discuss the benefits of nursing, and support efforts of nurses from other cultures to assimilate into nursing's culture.

The time to consider cultural and generational diversity is now. The nurse leader must consider the change in the population demographics, that industrialized nations are "graying" and the workforce is too. A survey of staff demographics can help the nurse leader prepare for an increase in chronic illness among the workforce as well as generational workforce issues and language and cultural challenges that might disrupt optimal effectiveness of operations (Kotlikoff & Burns, 2004).

Leveraging Diversity

Leveraging diversity is the ability of an organization to become culturally competent and, in doing so, value diversity from both a personal (the organization) and business (the customer base) perspective (Shipp & Davidson, 2001). This business strategy links the workforce, the workplace structure, and the marketplace, and displays the ability of organizations and their leaders to recognize and use every advantage to ensure success. Leveraging diversity maximizes all talents and intellectual capital within an organization and ensures that all persons are included in every aspect of the organization.

Leveraging diversity is known to boost employee morale, reduce grievances, and enhance problem-solving and decision-making abilities. This approach to management of human capital in an organization reduces barriers, enabling all employees to fully use their talents on behalf of the organization.

Leveraging diversity in the marketplace includes serving customer groups with a sensitivity to their cultures and allows an organization to maintain a multicultural perspective. Cultural diversity can be leveraged for bottom-line impact and therefore ties directly to business strategy and practices.

There are three leadership behavioral elements of leveraging diversity.

- The *cultural element* includes exerting influence within the organizational culture to set the tone for underlying values, beliefs, and principles.
- The *leadership element* includes giving employees a sense of direction, meaning, and purpose to navigate organizational waters as well as recognizing and using the full potential of all individuals in the organization.
- The *connectivity element* includes building a bridge between cultural and leadership elements and organizational intellectual capital, maintaining vision clarity, sharing power, and identifying and assessing problems.

The end result of leadership support and participation in leveraging diversity for an organization is an increase in productivity, efficiency, and quality and ultimately an improved work environment.

The nurse executive is a role model in setting the tone and direction of an organization's daily work effort. The nurse executive acts as a coach and supporter of all employees' work efforts to achieve the end goals and objectives of an organization.

Personnel Matters While Leveraging Diversity in the Workforce

While leveraging diversity in the workforce, there is overlap with human capital and human resources management functions. Areas to consider include writing and using objective documents, including job descriptions and performance appraisals. Leveraging diversity in the workplace should be a consideration during personnel selection efforts and orientation and training of new employees. Addressing behavioral issues and guiding employees to organizational support mechanisms such as employee assistance for alcohol, drug, or other issues are also times when leveraging diversity can increase an organization's productivity, efficiency, and quality, and ultimately lead to an improved work environment. Providing the assistance or the mechanism for employee assistance to all employees promotes increased productivity and leverages diversity.

Vulnerability audits and exit interviews offer opportunities to gather data about the work environment and consider whether this should be the time of change for job enrichment, engineering, rotation, or enlargement opportunities. Enhancing the work environment through job enrichment makes jobs more interesting and challenging, maximizes efficiency, and adds more variety to daily tasks. Goal-setting with employees provides objectives to structure the job while considering that job rotation adds variety (Slocum, 1981).

Organizational Transparency

Current management literature defines *organizational transparency* as a condition opposite secrecy in which there is a deliberate move away from opaqueness. A transparent organization encourages behaviors that support access to information, participation, and decision-making. These behaviors create a higher level of trust among all stakeholders.

Organizational transparency implies a trusting environment wherein transparency and trust are interconnected. Cultural trust in the organization requires clarity and consensus about what constitutes success, open access to information, and confidence in the competence of all involved. Leaders should consider creating an environment that fits the definition of success within the organization and for the organization.

Other important leadership behaviors include

- Practicing nonmanipulative leadership,
- Communicating frequently and repeating important information,
- Opening up access to documents regarding decisions,
- Sharing background information about important decisions,
- Providing clear financial reporting, and
- Hiring and appointing trustworthy people.

Challenges to organizational transparency include

- Risks from potential distortion of the truth through increased access to information,
- A slower-than-usual decision-making process, and
- Additional organizational vulnerabilities.

Organizational transparency does not guarantee that the right decisions are being made and may require additional time and resources at all organizational levels. Transparency may at some point have diminishing returns, when communication, information sharing, and trust levels reach a status quo and information flows in all directions. In the final analysis, the value of organizational transparency lies in the protection and promotion of an organization's reputation, a corporate culture of communication among all stakeholders, and the involvement of current and future members in decision-making processes (Fung, Graham, & Weil, 2007).

Nurse executives serve as role models and should support the organization's mission, promote communication in all directions, and participate in shared decision-making within the organization.

Lateral Violence

Lateral violence is aggressive and destructive behavior, in this case, of nurses against each other (Woelfle & McCaffery, 2007). The end result is damage to another's dignity, confidence, and self-esteem. Often, those who experience lateral violence in the workplace then transfer it to others.

Lateral violence in nursing can consist of a variety of behaviors, ranging from unintentional, thoughtless acts to purposeful, intentional, destructive acts meant to harm, intimidate, or humiliate a group or individual. Behaviors can range from random instances to a pattern, and such behaviors can create a hostile work environment.

Examples of behavioral lateral violence include

- Talking behind others' backs;
- Scapegoating;
- Criticizing a colleague in front of others;
- Excluding a coworker from group interaction;
- Withholding pertinent information;
- Violating a coworker's privacy and confidentiality;
- Making inappropriate, condescending remarks; and
- Displaying inappropriate nonverbal language, such as making faces or raising one's eyebrows.

Any time there exists an "us vs. them" attitude or when an imbalance of power occurs, conditions are prime for lateral violence. Examples of relationships in which lateral violence can occur include nurse manager to a staff nurse, nurse executive to a nurse manager or a staff nurse, nursing faculty member to a student nurse, and peer to peer.

The consequences of lateral violence can manifest themselves as physical symptoms, increased absenteeism and, in extreme cases, suicide of the targeted employee. Increased turnover of staff is also a symptom (Beecroft, Kunzman, & Krozek, 2001). Lateral violence can place patients at risk for poor care and outcomes. For example, what might happen to a patient when one nurse deliberately withholds pertinent information about the patient's care that needs to be shared with another nurse?

Nurse executives must be aware of and address lateral violence in the workplace and implement strategies to prevent and stop such behavior, such as

- Educating all staff and managers about this behavior;
- Disciplining any manager or staff member who engages in this behavior;
- Creating a culture that does not tolerate this behavior;
- Implementing organizational transparency, or having an open culture; and
- Implementing research to study this behavior in their own organizations.

The Health Work Environment

The *health work environment* is a topic that addresses nurses' working conditions, which are linked to the quality of care that is provided to patients and patients' safety. Accrediting organizations and Magnet include standards that address the working conditions because they are associated with health and safety outcomes for nurses and other healthcare providers (Geiger-Brown & Lipscomb, 2010). Employers are charged with a responsibility to assess and address the aspects of the nursing work environment that have been linked to hazards and adverse exposures for nurses and the most common health and safety outcomes of nursing work.

REFERENCES

Arrendondo, P. (1996). *Successful diversity management initiatives: A blueprint for planning and implementation.* Thousand Oaks, CA: Sage.

Beecroft, P. C., Kunzman, L., & Krozek, C. (2001). RN internship: Outcomes of a one-year pilot program. *JONA, 31*(12),575–582.

Bizony, N. (1999). Interest-based negotiation: Moving beyond our scarcity model. *OD Practitioner Online.* Retrieved from http://www.odnetwork.org/odponline/vol31n3/interestbased.html

Busche, G. D. (2007). Appreciative inquiry is not (just) about the positive. *OD Practitioner, 39*(4), 30–35.

Cooperrider, D. L., & Srivastra, S. (1987). Appreciative inquiry in organizational life. *Research in Organizational Change and Development, 1,* 129–169.

Covey, S. R. (2004). *The 7 habits of highly effective people.* New York: Free Press.

Epstein, D. G. (2003). Mediation, not litigation. *Nursing Management, 34*(10), 40–42.

Fisher, R., Ury, W., & Patton, B. (Eds.). (1991). *Getting to yes: Negotiating agreement without giving in.* New York: Penguin.

Fung, A., Graham, M., & Weil, D. (2007). *Full disclosure: The perils and promise of transparency.* New York: Cambridge University Press.

Geiger-Brown, J., & Lipscomb, J. (2010). The health care work environment and adverse health and safety consequences for nurses. *Annual Review of Nursing Research, 28,* 191–231.

Goleman, D. (1997). *Emotional intelligence.* New York: Bantam Books.

Goleman, D. (2000). *Working with emotional intelligence.* New York: Bantam Books.

Gottlieb, M., & Healy, W. J. (1998). *Making deals: The business of negotiating* (2nd ed.). Greenwich, CT: Communication Project.

Greer, E. (2006). *How to use the six laws of persuasion during a negotiation.* Cary, NC: Global Knowledge Training.

Higgs, M. (2006). *Beyond "high potential": Successful talent management.* Retrieved from http://www.google.com/url?sa=t&rct=j&q=&esrc=s&source=web&cd=6&ved=0CFMQFjAF&url=http%3A%2F%2Fwww.summit-events.com%2FDownloads%2FSuccessful_talent_management_Malcolm_Higgs.ppt&ei=860rUcaIPKe60AHY1YHwAg&usg=AFQjCNHtKQHyC_K-8GJxxCYn9wXUIAgShA&bvm=bv.42768644,d.dmQ

Huber, D. L. (2010). *Leadership and nursing care management* (4th ed.). St. Louis, MO: Saunders.

Marquis, B. L., & Huston, C. J. (2009). *Leadership roles and management functions in nursing.* Philadelphia: Wolters Kluwer/Lippincott Williams & Wilkins.

Kaplan, T. (1998). *The Tylenol crisis: How effective public relations saved Johnson & Johnson.* Retrieved from http://www.aerobiologicalengineering.com/wxk116/TylenolMurders/crisis.html

Katzenbach, J. R. (1997). The myth of the top management team. *Harvard Business Review, November–December,* 83–91.

Katzenbach, J. R., & Smith, D. (2003). *The wisdom of teams: Creating the high performance organization.* New York: McKinsey.

Kedia, S., & Burns, N. (1999). Global managers: Developing a mindset for global competitiveness. *Journal of World Business, 34*(3), 230–251.

Kinni, T. (2003). Exploit what you do best: The art of appreciative inquiry. *Harvard Management Update 8*(9). Available online at http://hbswk.hbs.edu/archive/3684.html

Kotlikoff, L. K., & Burns, S. (2004). *The coming generational storm: What you need to know about America's economic future.* Cambridge, MA: MIT Press.

Leveraging a diverse workforce. (n.d.). *BusinessWeek.* Retrieved from http://www.businessweek.com/adsections/diversity/diverselever.htm

Marquis, B. L., & Huston, C. J. (2009). *Leadership roles and management functions in Nursing: Theory and practice* (6th ed.). Philadelphia: Lippincott Williams & Wilkins.

Meyer, P. D. (2003, August). *The truth about transparency. Executive update.* Retrieved from http://www.asaecenter.org/PublicationsResources/EUArticle.cfm?ItemNumber=11786

Salovey, P., & Mayer, J. D. (1990). Emotional intelligence. *Imagination, Cognition, and Personality, 9,* 185–211.

Shipp, P. L., & Davison, C. J. (2001). Leveraging diversity: It takes a system. *Leadership in Action, 20*(6), 1–5. Retrieved from http://media.wiley.com/assets/51/56/jrnls_jb_lia_shipp.pdf

Slocum, J. W. (1981). Job Redesign: Improving the Quality of Work. *Journal of Experiential Learning and Simulation, 3,* 17–36.

Woelfle, C. Y., & McCaffrey, R. (2007). Nurse on nurse. *Nursing Forum, 42*(3), 123–131.

Yoder-Wise, P. S., & Kowalski, K. E. (2006). *Beyond leading and managing: Nursing administration for the future.* St. Louis, MO: Mosby.

CHAPTER 5

PROGRAM EVALUATION AND RESEARCH

PROGRAM EVALUATION

Models

Various models of program evaluation exist within the field of health care. The Joint Commission, which is discussed at greater length in Chapter 6, has long been regarded as the standard-bearer with regard to the evaluation first of acute care facilities, and more recently long-term care (LTC), specialty care, ambulatory care, and other healthcare entities. Joint Commission standards incorporate structure, process, and outcome evaluation.

The National Committee for Quality Assurance (NCQA) focuses on quality measures that show the degree of improvement in clinical practice, with a focus on evidence-based interventions. A 2002 NCQA report revealed that the quality of health care is improving, but also cautioned that there is still room for improvement. By its own calculations, NCQA estimated that more than 6,000 deaths and 22 million sick days could be avoided annually if identified "best practices" were more widely adopted.

NCQA's Health Plan Employer Data and Information Set (HEDIS) measures are used by employer groups and benefits managers to determine the comparative quality of particular health plans and health systems and to make recommendations to employees about their choice of health plan during the open enrollment period.

The National Database of Nursing Quality Indicators (NDNQI; see www.nursingworld.org/ResourcesForYou/NDNQI.aspx) is linked with the American Nurses Association's (ANA) Quality and Safety Initiative. Systematic data collection from more than 250 U.S. hospitals helps researchers determine how, if, or to what degree nursing affects patient outcomes. In addition to collecting patient care data, NDNQI also conducts a survey of nurse satisfaction (Taunton et al., 2004).

The National Forum for Healthcare Quality Measurement and Reporting (NQF; see http://www.qualityforum.org/), incorporated in 1999, is a not-for-profit, public–private collaborative created to develop and implement a national strategy for healthcare quality measurement and reporting. NQF's member groups work to promote a common approach to measuring healthcare quality and fostering systemwide capacity for quality improvement. The organization came into being as national trends demonstrated a decrease in quality patient outcomes and an increase in healthcare costs. Workforce productivity is integral to the improvement of quality and decreasing overall healthcare costs.

Performance Improvement/Continuous Quality Improvement/Total Quality Management

Performance improvement (PI) activities are now firmly embedded in the quality structure of most organizations, particularly those that seek Joint Commission accreditation. The plan–do–check–act (PDCA; see p. 24) cycle provides a model that is relatively easy to understand and able to graphically represent change over time in control charts. It provides a common language and a wide variety of tools to help all personnel engaged in the process.

The philosophy underlying *continuous quality improvement* (CQI) is to continually increase quality. As a particular goal is achieved and improvement sustained, the stakes are raised for that same goal. For example, if the baseline statistic for documentation of patient teaching consistent with the policies of the organization is 90%, and the long-term goal is 95%, perhaps the interim goal is 92%; followed the next year by 94%; and, finally, in the third year, if change is sustained, the bar is raised to 95%. Measurement continues until tools, techniques, and behavior patterns are part of daily practice for a period of months or years. Those involved with the project must then determine if the bar can be raised still higher, say to 98%, or if 95% is acceptable. In the latter situation, the staff would move on to another performance improvement initiative. The CQI process helps organizations focus on the "vital few" interventions that are likely to have the most applicability to health outcomes or to continued accreditation.

In organizations that embrace *total quality management* (TQM), everyone is committed to continuous improvement in her or his part of the organization. Although the impact of TQM in Japan, where it was developed, was astounding, the current world economy in developed countries does not reveal the "rosy" picture of a decade ago. A recessionary environment, including devaluation of the stock market, is taking its toll. Still, TQM's impact on productivity and quality is well documented (Barnard, 2009; Deming, 2000; Langley, Nolan, Provost, Nolan, & Clifford, 2009).

The Malcolm Baldrige National Quality Award was created to honor businesses that best exemplify commitment to TQM. The application process is intense and rigorous. In general, the businesses that originally competed for the Baldrige Award were industrial manufacturing or service organizations. More recently, healthcare-specific criteria were established. In 2002, the St. Louis–based SSM Health Care Organization became the first to win the coveted award for its exceptional service and achievements in the area of quality improvement (National Institute of Standards and Technology [NIST], 2002).

The American Nurses Credentialing Center's (ANCC's) Magnet Recognition Program®, initiated in 1994, also honors healthcare facilities and systems that "demonstrate sustained excellence in nursing care." There are currently 395 healthcare organizations in United States, and 4 international entities—2 in Australia, 1 in New Zealand, and 1 in Beirut, Lebanon—that were designated as Magnet facilities for their excellence in nursing service (ANCC, 2012).

Institutions that apply for Magnet status proceed through a rigorous evaluation process on the basis of quality indicators and standards of practice as defined in the ANA's (2009) *Nursing Administration: Scope and Standards for Practice.* Magnet status is awarded to an organization for a 4-year time period. Reapplication is as rigorous as the initial application and must demonstrate continued progression and improvement in all Magnet categories. Information on ANCC's Magnet Recognition Program can be obtained from www.nursecredenitaling.org/Magnet.

Outcomes Criteria

Stakeholder Satisfaction

Healthcare organizations have many stakeholders with a vested interest in their own satisfaction as well as in the perceived status of the organization. Not surprisingly, research has demonstrated a correlation between employee satisfaction and patient/client satisfaction.

Patient/Client and Family

Most organizations conduct patient satisfaction surveys to determine the perception of the services they provide to and for patients. Organizational leaders are sometimes surprised that their definition of "quality" and that of the patient/family differ. For example, suppose Hospital A has the best outcome for cardiovascular surgery (96%), but the perception of service on the most recent patient satisfaction survey is in the mid-range (76%). Suppose, on the other hand, that Hospital B falls 10 points short of Hospital A on surgical outcomes (86%), but far surpasses Hospital A on perception of services (97%).

Organizations conduct surveys of people in the community who do not use their services to determine if the perception of "strangers" is similar to or different from those familiar with the institution. The results of such surveys may be used in creating or revising the organization's marketing plan.

While well-meaning staff members and managers may conduct informal satisfaction surveys at the unit level, a word of caution is needed. The survey results that "count" are those that are derived from the use of valid, reliable survey instruments and processes. The Press Ganey Survey (Fullam, Garman, Johnson, & Hedberg, 2009; www.pressganey.com) is widely used by healthcare institutions throughout the United States.

Staff and Physicians

Organizations also periodically "take the pulse" of staff members and physicians. For some facilities, a high rate of physician satisfaction translates to an improved bottom line.

Results of staff satisfaction surveys identify areas of focus for managers who are interested in improving the workplace environment. Again, a word of caution is in order. Suppose there are 140 employees on a given unit who care for patients 7 days a week, 24 hours per day. All were given the opportunity to complete a satisfaction survey. A total of 12 surveys were returned, all of them from the night shift. The greatest source of dissatisfaction has to do with the hours of work. Those who responded to the survey indicated a preference for an 11:00 p.m. to 7:00 a.m. rotation rather than the midnight to 8:00 a.m. rotation that has been in place for several years. The manager most likely has a great deal more work to do before acting on this finding.

Payers

Payers, too, are stakeholders with a keen interest in the status of the organizations with which they contract. Payer satisfaction has to do with value for their investment and satisfaction by their employees with the care and service provided. Certainly payers are interested in the organization's quality outcomes, but benefit coordinators want to know that employees receive timely, high-quality care that keeps them well and productive in the job setting or healthy in their retirement.

Report Cards

Industry report cards issued by accrediting bodies such as those mentioned above or by private or quasi-governmental "watchdog" agencies are part of doing business in today's quality-conscious environment. Report cards compare facilities or organizations with one another or show how agencies compare with preestablished industry benchmarks.

Institutions that want to excel in the area of quality may wish to avail themselves of the tools and techniques offered by such organizations as the Institute of Healthcare Improvement (IHI; see http://www.ihi.org) and National Institute of Standards & Technology (NIST), specifically the Baldrige National Quality Program's Criteria for Performance Excellence (in Health Care; see http://www.quality.nist.gov/).

Benchmarking

Benchmarking is a technique that identifies "best in class" as a means of comparing one's practice or institution with those who are judged objectively to be the standard-bearer or pacesetter in a given category. For example, the Magnet hospital program highlights those institutions that meet or exceed the highest standards for patient care; outcomes of care; and staff retention, involvement, and satisfaction. Internal benchmarks may identify a particular department with a consistently excellent track record.

However, benchmark achievements often are published, and others are challenged or admonished to achieve the same outcomes as the benchmark company or department without benefit of learning about the *process* the facility went through to achieve its esteemed status. It is in learning about the process that people or institutions gain the most insight about what creates success for those that others hope to emulate.

Functional Status

Functional areas within the organization include production, marketing, distribution, human resources, marketing, finance, and research and development. The extent to which each functional unit accurately performs the work for which it is accountable, the better positioned the organization is to achieve its goals and surpass its competitors.

Functional areas are interdependent; a failure to achieve intended results in one area may cause problems in another area. For example, suppose the organization is known for its excellence in the care of patients undergoing invasive cardiovascular surgery. Marketing conducts an aggressive ad campaign at the same time 4 (of 11) of the most expert cardiovascular surgical nurses are planning to retire within the next 6 weeks with no replacements in sight despite the fact that human resources has been recruiting for months. Unless representatives of the various functional areas are in constant communication with one another and continually evaluate their overlapping strategies with an eye on the whole of the organization, minor or major calamities are inevitable.

HCAHPS

The Center for Medicare and Medicaid Services initiated the Hospital Consumer Assessment of Healthcare Providers and Systems (HCAHPS), which is "the first national, standardized, publicly reported survey of patients' perspectives of hospital care. HCAHPS (pronounced 'H-caps'), also known as the CAHPS® Hospital Survey, is a 27-item survey instrument and data collection methodology for measuring patients' perceptions of their hospital experience" (HCAHPS Hospital Survey, n.d.). HCAHPS ties to reimbursement for inpatient prospective payment system (IPPS) hospitals. Annual payment can be reduced by 2.0 percentage points if an IPPS hospital does not participate in the HCAHPS survey.

Performance Improvement Systems

Every organization implements its own type of performance improvement system. Some organizations utilize NDNQI; others utilize Lean Sigma Six. Some organizations implement programs such as the Plane Tree program as a method to improve patient care and satisfaction. Nurse executives need to be part of the executive team that selects the performance improvement system best suited for their respective organization.

RESEARCH

Conducting Research

Research is critical to the growth of any profession. Nurses should be able to use and understand research and statistical methods for the following reasons:

- To read the literature and studies with scrutiny and apply findings to their work,
- To conduct applied research relevant to patient needs,
- To move nursing from the artistic and intuitive toward the deliberative and tested so that care at the bedside is based on solid knowledge coupled with compassion, and
- To move nursing closer to the other applied health fields that are research-based and in this way develop more collaborative relationships with colleagues in other health-care disciplines.

Research can be categorized in the following manner:

- *Applied*: That which is designed to solve a practical problem or to answer an immediate question;
- *Basic:* That which is designed to test and evaluate theories or to contribute to a body of knowledge;
- *Case study:* That which involves intensive study or investigation of a single individual or group;
- *Descriptive:* That which describes or reports selected variables and seeks to prove (to others) that facts already accepted really exist (no hypotheses are tested);
- *Developmental:* That which deals with changes that occur as a result of maturation or development;
- *Experimental:* That in which participants are randomly assigned to experimental and control groups, an independent variable is manipulated, and scores on a dependent variable are measured, leading to conclusions about the effect of the independent variable on the dependent variable;
- *Field:* That conducted in the real world or in a natural setting;
- *Historical:* That which is designed to explain or interpret particular phenomena that have happened in the past;
- *Laboratory:* That which is conducted in a setting specifically designed for research;
- *Longitudinal:* That which involves measuring the same individuals at various times as they grow older; and
- *Qualitative:* That which does not follow the scientific model and that focuses on the collection and subjective interpretation of data rather than on the testing of a theory.

Data gathering is an important element of any research endeavor. Data are qualitative or quantitative:

- *Qualitative (words):* Descriptions in narrative form: concepts, facts, verbatim statements from participants, and subjective observations
- *Quantitative (numbers):* Enhances the precision of studies; data are categorized in the following ways:
    - *Nominal:* Data are categorical and cannot be arranged in any order with respect to one another. Examples include marital status and religious or political affiliation.
    - *Ordinal:* Data categories are ordered, but differences cannot be determined or are meaningless. Examples include socioeconomic status (e.g., lower middle, middle, upper middle classes), car sizes (e.g., compact, midsize, luxury), restaurant/hotel ratings (e.g., one star, five stars), or survey questionnaires in which respondents are asked to rank order selected choices.
    - *Interval/ratio:* Data have categories that are ordered; meaningful differences can be determined. With ratio data there is an absolute zero; with interval data there is no absolute zero. Ratio data are considered a subset of interval data. Examples of interval data include temperature, time (Gregorian calendar measurements), or survey questionnaires using known intervals (as with Likert-type scales). Examples of ratio data include age, weight, height, or distance. Ratio and interval data measure relationships or differences.

Instruments and methods used to gather data must be valid, reliable, and usable.

- *Validity* means that the data-gathering instrument measures what it is supposed to measure. It is the most important characteristic of a measuring device. Validity is never 100%, as something always falls short. However, it is important to determine if the validity of an instrument is sufficient to be used for the purpose of the particular study under investigation.
- *Reliability* means how well and how consistently an instrument measures something. Most instruments are not perfect, and their reliability is expressed as a coefficient number, with 1.00 equal to 100%. A correlation coefficient equal to or greater than .80 is considered an acceptable level of reliability. The degree of reliability is determined by the purpose for which the instrument is used.

An instrument may be *reliable* (able to measure something consistently) without being *valid* (appropriate instrument for the measures desired). However, an instrument may not be considered valid unless it has both reliability and validity; it must measure consistently and accurately what it is supposed to measure.

No matter how well the research question is formulated or the hypothesis generated, the outcome of a study depends on the appropriateness of measures used; their validity and reliability; and the extent to which effective, useful data analysis techniques can make the findings meaningful and useful for their intended purpose.

Pretesting, or conducting a pilot study, of self-developed instruments is essential. Evaluating the strengths and weaknesses of an instrument and making needed revisions ensures proper use of the data-gathering tool.

Study Population and Sampling

The term *population* is used to define the group to be studied.

- *Target:* Individuals or things that meet the criteria of interest to the investigator
- *Sample:* A miniature version of the target population; a group that is usually available for a study and who meet the criteria of the target population.

Sampling types include

- *Random:* All members of the population have an equal chance of being included in the study.
- *Probability:* The investigator can specify for each element of the population the probability that it will be included in the sample. Sample units are selected by chance, and neither investigator nor the population elements have any conscious influence on the constitution of the final sample. *Simple random, stratified random,* or *cluster* sampling are considered part of this category.
- *Non-probability:* The investigator has no ability to estimate the probability that each element of the population can or will be a part of the sample or even that it has a chance of being included. Non-probability samples do not permit generalization beyond the current study group. Confounding factors may influence this type of sampling more than a random sampling, thus making findings of less potential value to a broader population.
  - *Convenience:* Simply taking those people who are available in the right place at the right time *(accident sampling).*
  - *Purposive:* Investigator establishes certain criteria and selects participants according to these criteria *(judgment sampling).*
  - *Quota:* Similar to convenience sampling, but with controls to prevent overloading with participants having certain characteristics.

The *sample size* is determined by the number *(N)* that can logically be included; are available; and that suit the purpose of the study for precision, target population size, desirability for generalization beyond the study group, and importance of the outcomes for decision-making. It is generally wise to use a sample large enough to be representative of the target population and to use the largest group possible within the constraints of the study. In general, the larger the sample, the less error there is in measurement and the more significant the findings. An *N* of less than 30–45 participants reduces the ability to use strong, powerful statistical analysis of the data.

Correlation is the relationship between two or more factors or characteristics. Correlation is often spoken of as "positive" or "negative" in relation to a numerical coefficient. However, correlation of factors with one another in no way proves causation. Although cause-and-effect relationships often are implied, such assumptions can be erroneous and cannot be substantiated by statistical analysis.

Measures of Central Tendency and Dispersion

The mean, median, and mode are all measures of central tendency, the purpose of which is to isolate one response that is representative of the sample. In some cases, the three measures may be identical to one another.

- *Mean:* The average score of the sample; can be used with interval or ratio data. To find the mean, total the scores of the sample, then divide the total by the number of scores in the sample.
- *Median:* The point in the scale with half the total scores above the particular point and half the total scores below that point; can be used with ordinal data or any rating scale.
- *Mode:* The category that occurs with the greatest frequency; the only appropriate measurement for nominal data.

Dispersion, or the degree to which participants are distanced from the mean, is captured in a measure known as *standard deviation (SD).* This measure requires interval or ratio data. *SD* is described as the "average of the averages." It is the most stable measure of variability, that is, the measure of the distance from the mean. *SD* is a mathematical construct calculated by

- Computing the deviation of each raw score from the mean;
- Squaring and then summing the deviation scores;
- Dividing the sum by the number of scores *(N)* or by $N - 1$; and then
- Computing the square root of the sum.

A practical example is as follows (for illustrative purposes only; all subtleties of the mathematical model are not included here):

> Suppose there are 100 patients with diabetes who have had an HgbA1C blood test performed within the past month. The mean value of the HgbA1C test results is 7.5, with a range of 6–14.5. The care team wants to know the value of the *SD* and applies the formula. The *SD* is calculated as ± 1.5, which means that 68% of the patients have a HgbA1C that is 1 *SD* (1.5) from the mean, or 7.5 ± 1.5 (6.0 – 9.0). Another 28% have a HgbA1C that is 2 *SDs* (3.0) from the mean, or 7.5 ± 3.0 (4.5 – 10.5), and only 4% of patients in the study have HgbA1C readings that are 3 or more *SDs* from the mean. If the *SD* were smaller (e.g., 0.5), the "spread" would be narrower. Conversely, if the *SD* were larger (e.g., 2.0), the "spread" would be wider.

Hypothesis

The *hypothesis* is an educated guess. It is the researcher's statement of an expected outcome based on his or her rationale and the design of the study. Hypotheses need be present only in scientific research studies. Generally, there are independent and dependent variables in a hypothesis:

- *Independent variable:* Considered to be the cause; occurs first.
- *Dependent variable:* Considered to be the effect; depends on and occurs after the independent variable.

For example, the turnover rate for nurses is greater under authoritarian leadership:

  - *Turnover* is the dependent variable, as it is affected when the independent variable is added.
  - *Authoritarian* is the independent variable, as it affects (causes) the turnover rate.

Utilizing Findings

Nursing has been criticized for its failure to vigorously pursue research and to incorporate the findings from research into practice. Until recently, research in nursing was considered an academic endeavor, conducted by those with advanced degrees, and was seen as having little practical application. This mindset took hold despite the fact that Florence Nightingale is recognized as a pioneer in the field of health research and was the first woman to be elected a fellow of the Royal Statistical Society. The value of research in the practice setting is now known and is supported through the establishment of nursing research committees whose members include nurses from all educational backgrounds and from a variety of clinical areas.

Translating Research Into Practice

It is unfortunate that a significant number of healthcare and nursing interventions are not based on current evidence (Melnyk & Fineout-Overholt, 2011). Much of what has and is practiced is based on ritual. There is a major thrust in health care and nursing to base all interventions on evidence from the field. In essence, one reviews the research that has been conducted and critically analyzes such research to see if practice should be changed based on the findings. If so, then the practitioner translates the research into the practice setting.

The purpose of research is to learn more about the world around us and to contribute new knowledge to a growing body of knowledge. For research to happen, one must first pose a question that warrants research. For a practitioner to translate research into practice and thus base practice on current evidence, a practitioner also must have a question, and it is hoped that this question was researched and some evidence exists that supports a practice change.

Bernadette Melnyk and Evelyn Fineout-Overholt (2011) are leaders in evidence-based practice for nursing. These nurse–researchers define the term *PICO(T):*

- *P*atient, population, or patient population;
- *I*ntervention;
- *C*omparative intervention or comparative patient population;
- *O*utcome; and
- *T*ime that the project or study be implemented for.

Obviously, the idea of translating research into practice and to base practice on evidence is to improve the patient care outcome. The following is an example of a practice change based on current evidence:

> The question was: Would detox protocols make it easier on the medical and nursing staffs in providing detoxification medications to clients addicted to chemical substances? Thinking about it more and refining the question: Would detoxification protocols improve the care to patients? Further thought and revision of the question lead to: Would detox protocols based on current evidence improve care to patients?
>
> The first step was seeing what research was out there on the detoxification of patients. When this was accomplished, the decision was made to try to implement this in practice. A comparison group was needed to see if the detox protocols really worked. Applying the PICOT format, the following was conceived:
>
> - *P* = The patient population was adult patients admitted to an inpatient addictions treatment center who were actively being detoxified from chemical substances.

- *I* = The intervention was evidence-based detoxification protocols.
- *C*= The comparative intervention and group were adult patients admitted to an inpatient addictions treatment center who were being detoxified from chemical substances without being on an evidence-based detoxification protocol.
- *O* = The outcomes were clinical measurements in both groups (i.e., hypertension, seizures, need for adjusting the protocols, pain).
- *T* = The PICO was implemented for a 3-month period.

It was noted that the detoxification protocols improved patient care. A focus group of nurses was interviewed to see the impact on nursing, which was all positive.

The following provides an example of an evidence-based practice project implemented in an acute care hospital setting.

EVIDENCE-BASED INTERVENTIONS TO REDUCE MEDICATION ERRORS IN THE ACUTE CARE HOSPITAL ENVIRONMENT

Purpose of Study

The purpose of this project was to determine if implementing evidence-based interventions would decrease the number of interruptions incurred by nurses during the medication administration process with an outcome of decreased medication errors. Strategies to decrease interruptions included the following:

- Developing of a quiet zone for registered nurses by having these nurses wear an armband with the word QUIET written on the armband;
- Having the charge nurse and unit secretary manage phone calls for the nurse administering medications;
- Creating a quiet area for medication preparation; and
- Educating healthcare team members on the negative impact that interrupting the nurse during medication administration has on patient safety.

Background Information

The Institute of Medicine (IOM; 1999; 2001; 2003) has reported nearly 100,000 iatrogenic events that occur in healthcare facilities on an annual basis. Since 2003, the goal of the IOM is to decrease these iatrogenic events with a resultant increase of quality care provided to patients. Several studies have documented that communication is one of the major problems contributing to such negative patient outcomes. Studies document these adverse outcomes to patients result from medication administration by registered nurses. The Institute of Medicine's (IOM) first Quality Chasm report (1999), *To Err Is Human: Building a Safer Health System*, states that medication-related errors are a significant cause of morbidity and mortality; they accounted "for one out of every 131 outpatient deaths, and one out of 854 inpatient deaths" (p. 27). Medication errors are estimated to account for more than 7,000 deaths annually. When analyzed, there are multifactorial reasons as to why medication errors occur. Studies document that interruptions both in the preparation and administration of medications are a major factor. Noise is one of these factors that contribute to this problem.

Potter and colleagues (2005) examined the acute work environment of registered nurses. In this ethnographic qualitative study that employed a mixed methodological approach involving 7 staff registered nurse, Potter and colleagues noted that there are a high number of cognitive shifts and interruptions that add to a nurse's cumulative cognitive load, which creates interruptions in nurses performing interventions. Potter and colleagues particularly noted that such interruptions occur during medication preparation and administration. The authors concluded that attention must be given to how care systems and work processes complement or interfere with nursing's cognitive work.

Stratton and colleagues (2004) conducted a descriptive study that surveyed a convenience sample of 57 pediatric and 227 adult hospital nurses regarding medication errors reported on their units. This study examined why medication errors occur, and why medication errors are not always reported. This study primarily focused on pediatric data, with a comparison to adult acute care nurses. Pediatric nurses indicated that a higher proportion of errors were reported compared with adult nurses (67% compared with 56%). Medication error rates per 1,000 patient-days computed from actual occurrence data were also higher on pediatric (14.80) as compared with adult units (5.66). Distractions and interruptions as well as RN-to-patient staffing ratios were the major reasons medication errors occurred. The authors concluded that nurse administrators focus on individual nurses rather than the system. Such a focus on the individual nurse causes fear for that nurse, with a resultant decrease in the actual number of medication errors being reported. The authors recommend that the systems for medication administration rather than individual nurses are examined.

Hughes and Blegen (2005) conducted a meta-analysis of medication administration. The authors noted that the organizational climate as well as interruptions are major factors in medications being administered incorrectly. These authors also note that this problem is multifactorial in nature.

Question Guiding Inquiry (PICOT)

Healthcare team members have many opportunities to identify clinical problems surrounding their areas of practice. However, integration of a clinical question into a format that will yield the most relevant and best evidence is the first step of evidence-based practice (Melnyk & Fineout-Overholt, 2005, 2011).

So, do interventions targeted to decrease noise and other interruptions during medication administration by registered nurses in acute care medical-surgical units decrease medication error events?

Population (P):

- The target population was a diverse sample of registered nurses in two acute care hospital settings who administer medications on medical-surgical nursing units.

Intervention (I):

- Develop a quiet zone for registered nurses by having these nurses wear an armband with the word (QUIET) written on the armband.
- Have the charge nurse and unit secretary manage phone calls for the nurse administering medications
- Create a quiet area for medication preparation
- Educate healthcare team members on the negative impact that interrupting the nurse during medication administration has on patient safety.

Comparison (C):

- Medication error events were totaled for 2009 broken down by specialty area, i.e., critical care, obstetrics, medical-surgical, and emergency department. These data were compared to medication error events for a 3-month time period that the intervention was implemented. Medication error events also were compared between both hospital units participating in the study during the 3-month time period that the study was implemented.

Outcome (O):

- A decrease in the number of medication error events, which ultimately prevents adverse medication reactions and results in improved quality of care provided to patients.

Time (T):

- The study was implemented for a 3-month time period.

Summary of Study

This study did not involve research subjects nor interventions to research subjects.

This study was conducted during the months of August, September, and October, 2010.

For this 3-month time period, a quiet zone for nurses administering medications was created on two different similar nursing units in two divisions of a hospital system in New Jersey. MIDAS aggregate data, which are collected in an ongoing manner for all services at the hospital system by the Risk Management Department, were compared for the same time period in the prior year. It was noted that there were zero medication errors during the study time period at one of the nursing units at one of the hospital divisions for all 3 months of the study. There was a noted decrease of about 70% of reportable medication errors at the second hospital unit in the other hospital division during the same time period. Specific unit factors different at the second nursing unit compared to the first nursing unit could explain why the same rates were not achieved at both facilities.

Conclusions/Outcome

Creation of a quiet zone for the administration of medications at one of the hospital units demonstrated zero medication errors for the study time period.

A significant decrease in medication errors during the study time period was noted at the other hospital division. Unit-specific factors may explain why the rates were different at both facilities.

Decreased medication errors should have a positive effect on patient care outcomes.

The nursing research committee had recommended replication of this study in the fall of 2011 on different units at both hospital divisions to ascertain if the same results could be achieved; therefore, it was requested to keep this study open for an additional 1-year time period.

The replication of this study was never implemented because a major change in practice had been implemented both hospital divisions that could have significantly affected the results of the study. The hospital implemented a telephone system that would ring the nurse if a monitor alarm was not within set parameters. Nurses were being constantly rung by the telephone, so they saw no purpose in replicating the study. This was reported to the nursing research council.

Facilitating Research

Many organizations, even those without academic affiliation, now sponsor nursing research committees, provide assistance with grant writing, and educate staff about the value and process of research. Leaders should, to the extent possible, foster research in their institutions and thus contribute to nursing's growing body of evidence-based knowledge.

Writing Grants

Academic institutions and larger healthcare systems employ grant writers who are responsible for identifying sources of grants, skillfully crafting the grant proposal, and guiding it through the grant process. Workshops are available in most geographical locations or from reputable institutions through the Internet for those who would like to learn more about the process and the availability of grants.

Organizations sometimes offer small restricted grants that provide novice grant writers an opportunity to develop a modest research project and apply for funds to carry it out within their organizational setting.

Certain private charities, most notably the Pew Charitable Foundation and the Robert Wood Johnson Foundation, offer grants for a wide range of healthcare endeavors. The U.S. government underwrites millions of dollars in grants each year. Drug companies are exceedingly liberal in providing grant monies, so much so that an obligation to disclose association is now a requirement of any function that may be sponsored by these same companies.

Protection of Human Subjects

The protection of human subjects is of great concern to all of those involved in research. *Institutional review boards (IRBs)* exist to ensure that participants in research studies are protected from unethical practices and unscrupulous researchers.

Regulations in the Health Insurance Portability and Accessibility Act of 1996 (HIPAA, P.L. 104-191) governing research are of interest in a variety of settings. A comprehensive discussion of HIPAA rules that apply to research is beyond the scope of this text (see Chapter 6 for more information). HIPAA regulations add a layer of protection to the manner in which data produced by healthcare institutions can be accessed, analyzed, and reported. In addition, practitioners engaged in research must become fully aware of and comply with HIPAA regulations concerning privacy authorization (U.S. Department of Health and Human Services, 2003).

Ethical Conduct

The National Institutes of Health (NIH) requires all members of its 14 IRBs to successfully complete a computer-based training (CBT) program as part of their affiliation with NIH. NIH makes the CBT program available, at no charge, to others. Several healthcare organizations involved with human subjects' research take advantage of the availability of the CBT program for their own staff members. The program focuses on the clinicians' responsibility to remain above reproach when involved with research having to do with the health and welfare of those they have committed to serve (to access the NIH IRB course, visit http://www.nihtraining.com/ohsrsite/IRBCBT/intro.php; see Chapter 6 for more information on ethics).

SUMMARY

As nursing continues to advance as a discipline, it is vital that all nurses embrace research and translate the findings from research into everyday practice. Because nursing is a practice discipline, it is the patients who ultimately benefit from our interventions. Do you want to have care rendered to you based on ritual and what has been handed down from one generation of nurses to the next, or do you want care rendered to you based on the most current evidence in the field?

REFERENCES

American Nurses Association. (2009). *Scope and standards for nursing administration.* Silver Spring, MD: American Nurses Publishing.

American Nurses Credentialing Center. (2009). *Find a Magnet organization.* Retrieved from http://www.nursecredentialing.org/Magnet/FindaMagnetFacility.aspx

American Nurses Credentialing Center. (2012). *Magnet Recognition Program.* Retrieved from www.nursecredenitaling.org/Magnet

Barnard, C. (2009). *Performance improvement basics: A resource guide for healthcare managers* (2nd ed.). Marblehead, MA: HCPro.

Deming, W. E. (2000). *Out of crisis.* Cambridge, MA: MIT.

Fullam, F., Garman, A. N., Johnson, T., & Hedberg, E. (2009). The use of patient satisfaction surveys and alternative coding procedures to predict malpractice risk. *Medical Care. 47*(5), 553–559.

Health Insurance Portability and Accountability and Accessibility Act of 1996, P.L. 104-191, 110 Stat. 1936.

Gitlin, L. N., & Lyons, K.J. (2004). *Successful grant writing: Strategies for health and human service professionals.* New York: Springer Publishing.

Hospital Care Quality Information from the Consumer Perspective. (n.d.) *HCAHPS hospital survey.* Retrieved from www.hcahpsonline.org/home.aspx

Hughes, R. G., & Blegen, M. A. (2008). Medication administration safety. In R. G. Hughes (Ed.), *Patient safety and quality: An evidence-based handbook for nurses* (pp. 924–985). Rockville, MD: Agency for Healthcare Research and Quality.

Institute of Medicine. (1999). *To err is human: Building a safer health system.* Washington, DC: National Academy Press.

Institute of Medicine. (2007). *Preventing medication errors.* Washington, DC: National Academy Press.

Kohler, S., Rack, K., Davis, A., & Vi Naylor, D. (2006). Facilitators and barriers to 10 National Quality Forum safe practices. *Journal of Medical Quality, 21*(5), 323–334.

Langley, G. J., Nolan, T. W., Provost, L. P., Nolan, K. M., & Clifford, N. L. (2009). *The improvement guide: A practical approach to enhancing organizational performance.* San Francisco, CA: Jossey-Bass.

Melnyk, B. M., & Fineout-Overholt, E. (2005). *Evidence-based practice in nursing and healthcare: A guide to best practice.* Philadelphia: Lippincott Williams & Wilkins.

Melnyk, B. M., & Fineout-Overholt, E. (2011). *Evidence-based practice in nursing and healthcare: A guide to best practice* (2nd ed.). Philadelphia: Lippincott Williams & Wilkins.

Mulloch, K., & Porter O'Grady, T. (2010). *Introduction to evidence-based practice in nursing and health care.* Sudbury, MA: Jones and Bartlett.

National Database of Nursing Quality Indicators. (2009). *Home page.* Retrieved from https://www.nursingquality.org

National Committee for Quality Assurance. (2002). *The state of health care quality 2002: Industry trends and analysis.* Washington, DC: Author.

Newhouse, R., Dearholt, S., Poe, S., Pugh, L., & White, K. (2007). *Johns Hopkins nursing evidence-based practice model and guidelines.* Indianapolis, IN: Sigma Theta Tau International.

Polit, D. F., & Beck, C. T. (2011). *Essentials of nursing research: Appraising evidence for nursing practice* (8th ed.). Philadelphia: Lippincott Williams & Wilkins.

Potter, P., Boxerman, S., Grayson, D., Sledge, J. Dunagan, C. & Evanoff, B. (2005). Understanding the cognitive work of nursing in the acute care environment. *JONA, 35*(7/8), 327–335.

Taunton, R. L., Bott, M. J., Koehn, M. L., Miller, P., Rindner, E., Pace, K., et al. (2004). The NDNQI: Adapted index of work satisfaction. *Journal of Nursing Measurement, 12*(2), 101–122.

Stratton, K. M, Blegen, M. A., Pepper, G., & Vaughn, T. (2004). Reporting of medication errors by pediatric nurses. *Journal of Pediatric Nursing, 19*(6), 385–392.

U.S. Department of Health and Human Services. (2003). *Protecting personal health information in research: Understanding the HIPAA privacy rule.* Retrieved from http://privacyruleandresearch.nih.gov/pr_02.asp

LEGAL AND REGULATORY ISSUES; HUMAN CAPITAL; HEALTHCARE POLICY AND POLITICS; ETHICS

LEGISLATION

Americans with Disabilities Act of 1990: Revised 2008

President George H. W. Bush signed the Americans with Disabilities Act of 1990 (ADA; P.L. 101-336) into law on July 26, 1990. The act was designed to ensure that otherwise qualified individuals with disabilities enjoy the same employment opportunities as those without disabilities. Under the ADA, the term *disability* with respect to an individual has three distinct definitions: (1) a physical or mental impairment that substantially limits one or more major life activities, (2) a record of such impairment, or (3) being regarded as having such an impairment. An individual must satisfy at least one of these definitions to be considered an individual with a disability for the purposes of this act.

The Equal Employment Opportunity Commission (EEOC) published its final regulations implementing the equal employment provisions of the ADA on July 26, 1991. The ADA is organized into five titles:

- *Title I. Employment:* Prohibits employers from discriminating on the basis of an individual's disabilities and applies to all facets of employment, including application for employment and terms of employment.
- *Title II. Public Services:* Requires public entities employed in public transportation services to provide accessible services to people with disabilities.

- *Title III. Public Accommodations and Services Operated by Private Entities:* Prohibits discrimination in places of public accommodations provided by private entities, such as lodgings, restaurants, educational facilities, and so forth.
- *Title IV. Telecommunications Relay Services:* Requires carriers of telephonic services to provide equal communication opportunities to disables persons.
- *Title V. Provisions:* Provides certain miscellaneous provisions, including state immunity, attorney fees, and prohibition against employer retaliation.

Effective dates for Title I and Employment Provisions of Title I that most affect employers include

- For employers with 25 or more employees, July 27, 1992
- For employers with 15 or more employees, July 27, 1994.

Reasonable accommodation within the workplace is addressed within Title 1:

> No covered entity shall discriminate against a qualified individual with a disability because of the disability of such individual in regard to job application procedures; the hiring, advancement, or discharge of employees; employee compensation; job training; and other terms, conditions, and privileges of employment. (Americans with Disabilities Acts of 1990)

EEOC defines the term *reasonable accommodation* to mean the following:

- Modifications to the job application process that enable a qualified individual with a disability to be considered for the position,
- Modifications to the work environment or the manner or circumstances under which the position held or desired is customarily performed that enable a qualified person with a disability to perform the essential functions of that position, and
- Modifications that enable an employee with a disability to enjoy the same benefits and privileges of employment as those without disabilities.

The ADA generally adopts the enforcement provisions of Title VII of the Civil Rights Act of 1964, as amended (see below). The EEOC is the designated enforcement arm under both Title VII and the ADA.

Affirmative action differs from the EEOC in that it enhances employment opportunities for protected groups of people. Affirmative action refers to equal opportunity employment measures that federal contractors and subcontractors are legally required to adopt. An example would be the Vietnam Veterans Readjustment Act of 1974, whereby employers with government contracts must take steps to enhance the employment opportunities of disabled and other veterans of the Vietnam era. Affirmative action today continues to protect and enhance employment opportunities for groups and considers the factors of race, color, religion, gender, and national origin. Individual states have chosen to ban affirmative action to eliminate a quota system; examples are the California Civil Rights Initiative, Michigan Civil Rights Initiative, and Washington Initiative 200.

Rehabilitation Act of 1973

The Rehabilitation Act of 1973 (P.L. 93-112) also may legally affect some facilities. Section 504 of the act, merely one long sentence, provides that "No otherwise qualified handicapped individual in the United States ... shall, solely by reasons of his handicap, be excluded from the participation in, be denied benefits of, or be subject to discrimination under any program or activity receiving Federal Financial Assistance."

In general, this regulation prohibits employment discrimination against a qualified employee solely because of his or her disability. The thrust of the regulation is that employment decisions must be made without regard to physical or mental disabilities that are disqualifying. However, the requirements of the regulation go beyond mere "neutrality" and impose an obligation on the employer to take positive steps to hire and promote qualified individuals with disabilities. The regulations define a *qualified handicapped person* as one who "with reasonable accommodation, can perform the essential functions of the job in question" (Rehabilitation Act of 1973, P.L. 93-112). In other words, an employer may not insist that an employee with a disability perform all aspects or functions of a job, but only those that are "essential." The regulations comment that "handicapped persons should not be disqualified simply because they may have difficulty in performing tasks that bear only a marginal relationship to a particular job" (Rehabilitation Act of 1973, P.L. 93-112).

Another question raised by the regulations is what kinds of *reasonable accommodations* are required? The regulations require such accommodations to the physical or mental impairment of a applicant or employee with a disability unless the accommodation would impose "undue hardship" on the operation of the program. Enforcement of Section 504 is under the U.S. Office of Civil Rights of the U.S. Department of Health and Human Services. Removing barriers from a workplace provides the opportunity for reasonable accommodations. At some point, reasonable accommodations may infringe or inhibit operations, which would be the cause of undue hardship to the business operations, decreasing revenue and/or causing the business to fail.

Americans with Disabilities Act of 1990, Amended 2008

The 2008 amendment struck down lower court rulings on industry's inconsistent ADA accommodations to carry out the ADA's objectives of providing "a clear and comprehensive national mandate for the elimination of discrimination" and "clear, strong, consistent, enforceable standards addressing discrimination" by reinstating a broad scope of protection to be available under the ADA (Americans with Disabilities Act, available at http://www.ada.gov/pubs/ada.htm).

Three key strategies to successfully navigate the ADA:

- Delineate "mandatory" functions of job.
- Make the work environment handicapped accessible (remove barriers).
- Prepare job descriptions before advertising or interviewing applicants for the job.

Age Discrimination and Employment Act

Congress enacted Age Discrimination and Employment Act (ADEA; P.L. 90-202) in 1967; its purposes are to "promote employment of older persons based on their ability rather than age; to prevent arbitrary age discrimination in employment; to help employers and workers find ways of meeting problems arising from the impact of age on employment" (Age Discrimination in Employment Act of 1967). The *older persons* who are protected by the act are individuals who are at least age 40 but younger than age 65. In early 1978, the ADEA was amended to increase the protected upper age to 70 beginning January 1, 1979.

The ADEA serves two primary functions: (1) It prohibits arbitrary age discrimination in employment, and (2) it promotes employment based on ability. In this sense, it is similar to Title VII of the Civil Rights Act. Under the ADEA, it is unlawful to "fail or refuse to hire or to discharge any individual with respect to his compensation, terms, conditions, or privileges of employment, because of such individual's age" (Age Discrimination in Employment Act of 1967, P.L. 90-202, 81 Stat. 602). Age does not mean that employers cannot differentiate between employees or prospective applicants when hiring, firing, or promoting. The purpose of ADEA was not to lower performance standards or to make employers ignore differences in qualifications. What the statute requires is that the employer not differentiate solely on the basis of age.

Family Medical Leave Act, 1993, Revised 2008

The Family Medical Leave Act (FMLA) entitles employees to take reasonable leave for medical reasons; for the birth or adoption of a child; and for the care of a child, spouse, or parent who has a serious health condition. Employers must provide employees with leave for serious illness or family issues while maintaining insurance and equal position within the organization.

The 2008 amendment reads: "[T]o accomplish the purposes…in a manner that, consistent with the Equal Protection Clause of the Fourteenth Amendment, minimizes the potential for employment discrimination on the basis of sex by ensuring generally that leave is available for eligible medical reasons (including maternity-related disability) and for compelling family reasons, *on a gender-neutral basis*" (The Family and Medical Leave Act of 1993, as amended; emphasis added).

This complex law, with overlap and interaction between the ADA and FMLA, challenges nurse leaders with a need to work closely with the human resources department in executing the provisions of the law.

Civil Rights Act of 1964

The cornerstone of equal employment opportunity is a section of this act known as Title VII, the Civil Rights Act of 1964 (P.L. 88-352), which has had an impact on a wide range of employment practices from advertising, application forms, interviews, employment testing, and hiring procedures to wage and salary structures, fringe benefits, promotion, and seniority systems. Title VII prohibits discrimination because of race, color, religion, sex, national origin, handicap, age, or sexual preference. The thrust of Title VII is twofold: (1) It prohibits discrimination based on factors not related to job qualifications, and (2) it promotes employment based on ability and merit.

The law was developed to address discriminatory practices with respect to African Americans and was amended before its first passage to also protect women of all races. In addition, the law seeks to correct past injustices and sources of institutional job bias through mechanisms such as *affirmative action.* Title VII, as amended and strengthened by legislation in 1972 (The Equal Employment Opportunity Act of 1972, P.L. 92-261), was the culmination of the struggle of several decades to prohibit racial discrimination by private employers. There was no congressional legislation protecting the civil rights of employees prior to the 1960s; in that decade, Congress enacted several major laws to remedy that.

The guiding principle behind Title VII is that persons be considered on the basis of individual capacities and not on the basis of any characteristics generally attributed to the group. Also, those individual capacities must be related to the job to be performed and must not be for the purpose of "screening out" certain individuals. The underlying assumption of Congress is that the factors of race, color, sex, religion, age, sexual preference, disability, or national origin are never criteria in making employment decisions, except in certain limited situations.

While Title VII prohibits a wide variety of discriminatory activities, it does contain several significant exceptions. One permits discrimination based on sex, religion, or national origin in cases in which those factors constitute a bonafide occupational qualification (BFOQ), such as weight bearing mobility challenges such as stairs, or other physical challenges that become more difficult or unattainable with age. Where such a BFOQ is shown to exist, an employer may consider these factors in employment-related decisions.

To determine if discrimination practices exist in an organization, first an employee must determine if he or she is protected from discrimination under the law (exceptions include independent contractors, unpaid volunteers, and non-citizens employed overseas by U.S. employers). A second factor to consider is if the employer is subject to anti-discrimination laws (exceptions include employers with 15 or fewer employees, labor organiations, joint labor–management committees controlling job training programs). A third factor is whether the employer's conduct by law is considered discriminatory. A final factor is what grounds an employer might use to be discriminatory in hiring practices (Civil Rights Act of 1964).

Civil Rights Act of 1991

On November 21, 1991, President George H. W. Bush signed into law and made effective the Civil Rights Act of 1991 (P.L. 102-66). Aside from reversing seven U.S. Supreme Court decisions regarding employment discrimination, the law allows for compensatory punitive damages and the right to a jury trial when such damages are sought. Victims of intentional discrimination based on sex, religion, or disability may receive significant damage awards (between $50,000 and $300,000, depending on the size of the workforce). The law also provides for technical assistance and employee training.

Equal Employment Opportunity Commission and Affirmative Action

Equal employment laws deal with aspects of discrimination and employment because of race, color, religion, national origin, age, sex, pregnancy, sexual harassment, or sexual orientation. The Equal Employment Opportunity Commission (EEOC) is responsible for enforcing Title VII of the Civil Rights Act of 1964 (see above). It has issued guidelines for the act's interpretation and decides cases brought to it by individuals and groups who believe that they have experienced discrimination. EEOC lawsuits are brought on behalf of both individuals and groups and are filed under various statutes enforced by the Commission, including Title VII, ADA, the Age Discrimination Act of 1967 (ADEA), and Equal Pay Act.

The investigatory responsibility of the EEOC is broad. When it finds reasonable cause that a charge of discrimination is justified, the agency attempts to reach an agreement through persuasion and conciliation. If these efforts fail, the EEOC is empowered to bring a civil action against the employer. The lawsuit does not have to be filed by any particular person or persons, but may be on behalf of persons claiming to be aggrieved. Thus, a lawsuit brought by the EEOC could be initiated without specific employee complaints (generally, however, a specific complaint is made). When discrimination is found, courts have ruled that simply providing equal employment opportunity in the future is not enough.

The employer in some instances must "make whole" and "restore the rightful economic status" of all those in the affected class. Courts have the power to order any relief thought to be appropriate, which may include reinstatement or promotion of employees, with or without back pay. Although back pay liability is limited to the 2 years preceding the filing of the charge with EEOC, some back pay awards, including class action suits, have been extraordinarily expensive.

Sexual Harassment

Sexual harassment is a form of illegal discrimination that is broadly defined as the unwelcome sexual conduct on the part of a supervisor, coworker, or client. Two types of sexual harassment are most commonly identified in the workplace:

- *Quid pro quo:* Denied promotion or other work-related benefit because of refusal of sexual demands
- *Hostile work environment:* Sexually based conduct in the environment that is unwelcome and so pervasive that it changes the work environment, even if the employee is not the actual target of the conduct (EEOC: Sexual Harassment)

Employers are encouraged to take steps necessary to prevent sexual harassment from occurring. There should be clear communication to employees that sexual harassment will not be tolerated. Employers can educate their employees by providing sexual harassment training that increases awareness of the seriousness of the issue in the environment. Employers should also ensure that there is an effective complaint or grievance process in place and ensure immediate and appropriate action when an employee complains.

Corporate Compliance

Corporate compliance for healthcare organizations originally pertained to ethics within organizations and originated in nursing homes to ensure ethical billing practices to avoid Medicare and Medicaid fraud. Current operations require compliance with fraud and abuse laws and other federal/state regulatory laws for lawful behavior and corporate success. Most organizations appoint a corporate compliance officer and mandate education of all staff. The concept of *corporate compliance* mandates reporting of any act deemed illegal or unethical in nature to corporate compliance officers.

The Dodd-Frank Wall Street Reform and Consumer Protection Act of 2010 established a new Consumer Financial Protection Bureau. The mission of this act is to make markets for consumer financial products and services work for every American to detect and prevent financial fraud. The program is commonly referred to as the Whistleblower Program or Act.

The Whistleblower Program or Act includes provisions that cover:

- Eligibility of a disclosure
- Eligibility of a whistleblower
- Anti-retaliation provisions

The rules prohibit employers from interfering with the efforts of whistleblowers to disclose information. Employees who report violations internally to their employer can receive protection, can receive a reward, and are protected by law.

Fair Labor Standards Act

The Fair Labor Standards Act (FLSA; P.L.99-239) establishes minimum wage, overtime pay, record-keeping, and youth employment standards affecting full-time and part-time workers in the private sector and in federal, state, and local governments. There are few federal laws that have as profound an impact on business operations as this act. More than 85% of all non-supervisory employees are now covered by this act, which has been frequently amended by Congress since the first federal minimum wage was established at 25 cents an hour in 1938.

The Wage and Hour Division administers and enforces FLSA with respect to private employment; state and local government employment; and federal employees of the Library of Congress, U.S. Postal Service, Postal Rate Commission, and the Tennessee Valley Authority. The FLSA establishes a minimum wage below which no covered employee may be legally employed. However, the law sets a maximum number of hours in any week beyond which a person may be employed only if paid an overtime rate. A *workweek* is defined as a regularly reoccurring period of 168 hours in the form of 7 consecutive 24-hour periods.

The FLSA requires that minimum wage and overtime compensation payments must be made in cash or by check. The sole exception is that costs of board, lodging, and certain other facilities furnished to employees may be deducted from the cash amount paid. Applicable minimum wages must be paid for all hours worked and that the hours be added to ascertain whether overtime pay should be awarded.

In general, *hours worked* includes all the time an employee is required to be on duty on the employer's premises or at a prescribed workplace and all the time the employee is required or permitted to work for the employer. Note that work that is voluntarily performed (such as occurs when an employee remains longer than the prescribed work period to complete an assigned task) is included within the computation of hours worked. Thus, it is the duty of the employer who does not want to pay for this type of "extra" work to make sure that the employee concludes his or her work at the end of the assigned work period. The FLSA also includes specific regulations concerning issues such as waiting time; oncall time; preparatory and concluding activities; and attendance at lectures, meetings, training programs, and the like.

A record must be kept of hours worked each workday and each workweek. Any method of keeping time records is acceptable as long as it is accurate and shows all hours worked. Time clocks are a good means of recording work hours, but they are not required. Rounding to the nearest fraction of an hour (e.g., nearest 5 minutes, one-tenth or one-fourth) is permitted based on the rationalization that this agreement averages out over a period of time so that employees are fully paid for all hours they work.

The FLSA does not limit the number of hours in a day or days in a week an employee may be required or scheduled to work, including overtime hours, if the employee is at least 16 years old. The number of hours in a day or days in a week are for agreement between the employer and the employees or their authorized representatives. The FLSA has no provisions regarding the scheduling of employees, with the exception of certain child labor provisions. Therefore, an employer may change an employee's work hours without giving prior notice or obtaining the employee's consent (unless otherwise subject to a prior agreement between the employer and employee or the employee's representative, such as a labor contract; U.S. Department of Labor, n.d.b).

Overtime pay requirements also are provided for in the FLSA. Unless specifically exempted, employees covered by the FLSA must receive overtime pay for hours worked in excess of 40 hours in a workweek at a rate of not less than time and one-half of their regular rate of pay, which may be more but not less than the statutory minimum. Note that in this instance state regulations are more restrictive than FLSA regulations, and therefore, state rules relative to payment of overtime for 8 hours in one workday prevail. The regular rate includes all remuneration for employment except reimbursement for expenses incurred on the employer's behalf; premium payments for overtime work; discretionary bonuses, gifts, and payments in the nature of gifts; and payments for occasional periods when no work is performed due to vacation, holiday, or illness.

The FLSA does not require breaks or meal periods be given to workers. Some states may have requirements for breaks or meal periods. For workers in states that do not require breaks or meal periods, these benefits are a matter of agreement between the employer and the employee (or the employee's representative).

Exempt vs. nonexempt employees: Certain employees in an executive, administrative, professional, or outside sales capacity are considered exempt from both minimum wage and overtime pay.

Learners, apprentices, students, and persons subject to child labor regulations also are subject to exemption. Areas that must be considered in evaluating for exempt status include:

- Salary level (e.g., minimal salary, annual salary, prorated pay)
- Salary basis (e.g., predetermined pay received regularly)
- Job duties (duties, department, supervision of 2 or more employees; The Fair Labor Standards Act of 1938, as amended)

Whether an employee is exempt depends on his or her duties and responsibilities and the salary paid. Administrators should note that titles do not make an employee exempt, nor does the fact that he or she is paid a salary rather than on an hourly basis.

The areas of overtime compensation, record-keeping, and exemption status are the three most prevalent portions of the FLSA violated by facilities. Administrators must pay attention to the proper payment of overtime, the adequate record-keeping provisions, and the verification of exempt status of all employees not being paid overtime.

FLSA Child Labor Provisions

Child labor provisions state that the basic minimum age for employment is 16 years. Employment of 14- and 15-year-old youths is permissible but is limited to certain occupations, outside of school hours only, and under specified conditions of work as set forth in the regulations. Healthcare administrators are encouraged to pay particular attention to the child labor provisions especially as they relate to the casual employment of schoolchildren younger than age 16.

FLSA Amendments of 1989

On November 29, 1991, the U.S. Department of Labor's Wage and Hour Division issued a final rule allowing employers to require employees lacking basic skills to spend up to 10 hours in remedial training in addition to their 40-hour workweek without having to pay time and one-half for the overtime (FLSA Amendments of 1989, P.L.101-157). The exemption is limited to those employees who lack a high school diploma or whose reading or basic skills are at or below the 8th-grade level. Employers must keep records of the time spent in remedial education and amounts paid, which must be at their regular rate of pay. The training must be conducted during a set time and should be away from the employee's regular workstation. The training should be designed to provide reading and basic skills equivalent to the 8th-grade level.

A comprehensive FLSA presentation is available through the U.S. Department of Labor at **http://** www.dol.gov/compliance/laws/comp-flsa.htm#overview (scroll down to E-Tools and click on the PowerPoint link).

Equal Pay Act of 1963

The Equal Pay Act of 1963 (EPA; P.L. 88-38) was amended the FLSA to require that men and women performing equal work receive equal compensation. The EPA prohibits discrimination on the basis of gender in wage rates between employees performing work in jobs that require equal skill, effort, and responsibility that are performed under similar working conditions when in the same establishment (U.S. Equal Employment Opportunity Commission, n.d.).

Occupational Safety and Health Administration

The Occupational Safety and Health Administration (OSHA) covers any employer engaged in a business affecting commerce, requiring that employer to "furnish to each of his employees a place of employment which is free from recognized hazards that are causing, or are likely to cause death or serious physical harm" (U.S. Congress, Senate, Committee on Labor and Human Resources). Broadly written federal legislation, the Occupational Safety and Health Act of 1970 (P.L. 91-596) was modeled after the California (Cal–OSHA) program that was in effect before the establishment of the federal plan. The act has been amended several times since its inception.

OSHA is authorized to conduct workplace inspections on every business covered by the act. Obviously, it is impossible for the U.S. Department of Labor, the federal department in which OSHA resides, to inspect every entity covered by the law. Thus, OSHA inspections are generally conducted at the request of the employer (to verify potentially unsafe conditions) or in response to a complaint from an employee. According to OSHA, reporting priorities are assessed in the following order:

> Top priority are reports of imminent dangers—accidents about to happen; second are fatalities or accidents serious enough to send 3 or more workers to the hospital. Third are employee complaints. Referrals from other government agencies are fourth. Fifth are targeted inspections—such as the Site-Specific Targeting Program, which focuses on employers that report high injury and illness rates, and special emphasis programs that zero in on hazardous work such as trenching or equipment such as mechanical power presses. Follow-up inspections are the final priority. (OSHA, 2007)

Since the agency was created in 1971 with the goal of reducing workplace injuries and deaths, "occupational deaths have been cut by 62%, and injuries have declined by 42%" (OSHA, 2007). Worksite Voluntary Protection Programs (VPP) report lost workday cases as high as 60% to 80% lower than their industry averages. These reports have been verified by OSHA (2007). A reduction of lost workdays can result in increased worker protection, decreased business costs, enhanced productivity, and improved employee morale.

Record-keeping is required to verify compliance with the act. OSHA forms are supplied to employers for this purpose and are now available through the Internet. About 1.5 million employers with 11 or more employees—20% of the establishments that OSHA covers—must keep records of work-related injuries and illnesses. Workplaces in low-hazard industries such as retail, service, finance, insurance, and real estate are exempt from record-keeping requirements. Healthcare organizations are not among the exempted employers.

OSHA offers three cooperative plans to increase safety in the workplace. The Alliance Program works with employers, labor unions, trade or professional groups, and educational institutions interested in workplace safety and health. In collaboration with OSHA, the interested partners work toward prevention of injuries and illnesses in the workplace.

The Strategic Partnership Program is for employers with varied backgrounds, experience, and records in job safety and health who share a common commitment to improving workplace safety and health. VPPs serve as models of excellence for others in their industries and communities and are designed to recognize workplaces with excellent safety and health programs. VPPs are exempt from routine OSHA inspections.

There are two major types of laws in the field of occupational health and safety: (1) *preventive* and (2) *compensatory.* OSHA is an example of preventive law. Well-known compensatory laws that have been enacted are those for workers. Under workers' compensation, an employee who is injured or becomes ill as a result of a condition on the job is compensated for that injury, including reimbursement of medical and hospital costs, whether his or her own acts caused or contributed to causing the injury.

Health Insurance Portability and Accountability Act of 1996

The Health Insurance Portability and Accountability Act of 1996 (HIPAA, also known as Kennedy–Kassenbaum; P.L. 104-191) covers the electronic exchange and protection of healthcare data and has generated controversy ever since its passage. Title I of the law allows persons to qualify immediately for comparable health insurance coverage when they change their employment relationships. There is little disagreement with the "goodness" of this element of the law.

Title II of the law gives the U.S. Department of Health and Human Services the authority to mandate the use of standards for the electronic exchange of healthcare data; to specify what medical and administrative code sets should be used within those standards; to require the use of national identification systems for healthcare patients, providers, payers (or plans), and employers (or sponsors); and to specify the types of measures required to protect the security and privacy of personally identifiable healthcare information. As of April 2003, healthcare systems are required to show evidence of compliance with the intent of the law as it pertains to the exchange of data and the notification of such exchange.

There is no simple explanation for the intricacies of HIPAA. It is safe to say that healthcare administrators will be involved with the implementation and interpretation of its privacy rules for years to come. Whether the safeguards of personal health status information promised to the public through the enactment of HIPAA will be realized as intended is yet to be determined.

Omnibus Budget Reconciliation Acts

Congress passed the landmark Consolidated Omnibus Budget Reconciliation Act (COBRA; P.L. 99-272) health benefit provisions in 1986. The law amends the Employee Retirement Income Security Act (ERISA), the Internal Revenue Code, and the Public Health Service Act to provide continuation of group health coverage that otherwise might be terminated.

COBRA contains provisions giving certain former employees, retirees, spouses, former spouses, and dependent children the right to temporary continuation of health coverage at group rates. This coverage, however, is available only when coverage is lost due to certain specific events. Group health coverage for COBRA participants is usually more expensive than health coverage for active employees, because usually the employer pays a part of the premium for active employees, while COBRA participants generally pay the entire premium themselves. However, COBRA is ordinarily less expensive than individual health coverage.

The law generally covers group health plans maintained by private-sector employers with 20 or more employees in the prior year, employee organizations, or state or local governments. The law does not, however, apply to plans sponsored by the federal government and certain church-related organizations.

Group health plans sponsored by private-sector employers generally are welfare benefit plans governed by ERISA and subject to its requirements for reporting and disclosure, fiduciary standards, and enforcement. ERISA does not establish minimum standards or benefit eligibility for welfare plans or mandate the type or level of benefits offered to plan participants.

The original health continuation provisions were contained in Title X of COBRA. Provisions of COBRA covering state and local government plans are administered by the U.S. Department of Health and Human Services. From September 1, 2008, through February 16, 2009, those with a qualifying event of involuntary termination of employment may be eligible for an additional election opportunity under the American Recovery and Reinvestment Act of 2009 (ARRA; see below).

There are three elements to qualifying for COBRA benefits: (1) specific criteria for plan coverage, (2) qualified beneficiaries, and (3) qualifying events.

Plan Coverage

Group health plans for private-sector employers with 20 or more employees on more than 50% of its typical business days in the previous calendar year are subject to COBRA. Both full- and part-time employees are counted to determine whether a plan is subject to COBRA. Each part-time employee counts as a fraction of an employee, with the fraction equal to the number of hours that the part-time employee worked divided by the hours an employee must work to be considered full-time.

Qualified Beneficiaries

Qualified beneficiaries generally are individuals covered by a group health plan on the day before a qualifying event who is an employee or the employee's spouse or dependent child. In certain cases, a retired employee and his or her spouse and dependent children may be qualified beneficiaries. In addition, any child born to or placed for adoption with a covered employee during the period of COBRA coverage is considered a qualified beneficiary. Agents, independent contractors, and directors who participate in the group health plan also may be qualified beneficiaries.

Qualifying Events

Qualifying events are those that would cause an individual to lose health coverage. The type of qualifying event will determine the status of qualified beneficiaries and the amount of time that a plan must offer the health coverage to them under COBRA. For employees, qualifying events include

- Voluntary or involuntary termination of employment for reasons other than gross misconduct, and
- Reduction in the number of hours of employment.

For spouses, qualifying events include

- Voluntary or involuntary termination of the covered employee's employment for any reason other than gross misconduct,
- Reduction in the hours worked by the covered employee,
- Covered employee becoming entitled to Medicare,
- Divorce or legal separation of the covered employee, and
- Death of the covered employee.

For dependent children, qualifying events include

- Loss of dependent child status under the plan rules,
- Voluntary or involuntary termination of the covered employee's employment for any reason other than gross misconduct,
- Reduction in the hours worked by the covered employee,
- Covered employee becoming entitled to Medicare,
- Divorce or legal separation of the covered employee, and
- Death of the covered employee (U.S. Department of Labor, n.d.a).

Revision of COBRA in the American Recovery and Reinvestment Act of 2009

ARRA (P.L.111-05) of 2009 provides a premium reduction to certain qualified individuals and expanded eligibility for COBRA. Individuals who are eligible for COBRA coverage because of their own or a family member's involuntary termination of employment that occurred from September 1, 2008, through December 31, 2009, and who elect COBRA may be eligible to pay a reduced premium amount that is only 35% of the premium costs for COBRA coverage for up to 9 months.

HUMAN CAPITAL AND ORGANIZATIONS

Human capital can best be explained in the context of both an organizational and personal perspective. From the organizational perspective, *human capital* is:

- A group's collective knowledge, skills, and abilities
- Beliefs that investment in professional development and education will have a future return on investment.

From the personal perspective, human capital is personal attributes that are productive in some economic context (About.com-Economics, 2009).

The Importance of Human Capital Management

Knowledgeable and competent employees are the greatest asset of any organization. An organization is only as good as its people. *Human capital management* (HCM) fosters a positive work environment. Successful HCM and leadership promote employee engagement, employee motivation, employee development, and employee retention.

Human Capital and Human Resources

Human resource management is an integral part of HCM in supporting the organization's operations. Human resource functions include:

- Recruitment of new employees
- Incentives and compensation packages
- Organizational compliance with laws and regulations
- Setting day-to-day objectives necessary for streamlining activities within the organization to ensure that work is not done haphazardly (Hyde & Cook, 2004).

Compensation and Employee Benefits

The role of compensation and employee benefits in human capital management rewards and recognizes an organization's best employees and can be an effective recruitment tool. Effective strategies raise productivity and have a positive effect on the bottom line.

Compensation is the total amount of the monetary and non-monetary pay provided to an employee by an employer in return for work performed as required. Part of compensation, in addition to salary, is an employee benefits package, standard in organizations and expected by employees. Employee benefits packages generally consists of paid time off, health and life insurance, dental and vision insurance, paid prescriptions, flexible spending accounts, and long- and short-term disability insurance (About.com: Employee Benefits Packages, 2012).

Employee Satisfaction

Employee satisfaction can be defined as "the terminology used to describe whether employees are happy and contented and fulfilling their desires and needs at work.... [It] is a factor in employee motivation, employee goal achievement, and positive employee morale in the workplace" (Healthfield, 2012).

Certain factors contribute to employee satisfaction. They include:

- Positive management and leadership that supports a framework of goals, measurements, and expectations
- Treating employees with respect
- Providing regular employee recognition
- Empowering employees
- Offering a competitive package of benefits and compensation
- Providing employee company activities.

Common measures of employee satisfaction are used to monitor and provide opportunities to respond to workplace challenges. They include employee satisfaction surveys and small focus groups that focus on:

- Management and leadership
- Understanding of mission and vision
- Empowerment
- Teamwork
- Communication
- Coworker interaction.

Employee Rights

Employee rights can best be summarized in a review of the legal and regulatory issues that promote a safe and effective work environment. Employee rights can be summarized as the right to:

- A safe workplace (OSHA)
- Safe and healthful working conditions (OSHA)
- Participate in activities to ensure their protection from job hazards (OSHA)
- Receive protection from discrimination under whistleblower protection laws when using reporting provisions
- Be paid a minimum wage (FLSA)
- Be provided (in most cases) regular breaks, overtime pay, workers' compensation insurance, unemployment insurance, and time off under FMLA (in most cases)
- Work in an environment protected from sexual harassment (EEOC)
- Work in an environment that permits performance of essential functions of the job (ADA).

Recruitment Strategies

To meet an organization's goals of sustainability and profitability, it is necessary to attend to the personnel needs to operate efficiently and optimally. A general rule of thumb is to plan to hire for today's need and tomorrow's vision. Begin with determining the need to maintain the status quo or whether it is time for a change based on the work to be done. Have the demographics of the organization changed so that needs to be consideration or time for a job redesign?

In seeking to fill the personnel pipeline, leaders should consider internal candidates first. The advantages of recruiting internal candidates include having knowledge of the organization and culture, a network of interpersonal relationships with inside information, and access to channels for informal communication. Succession planning for nurse executives is a competency of accrediting bodies and professional organizations as a method to prepare for the future, support leadership positions that open in the organization, and recognize the value of internal leadership programs.

Proven recruitment approaches, depending on the time and need of an organization, include:

- Advertisement and social media networking
- Conference and trade shows
- Employee personal networks
- Healthcare industry contacts, professional organizations
- Organization's website
- Being an employer of choice.

Coaching, Mentoring, and Precepting

Coaching employees begins at the point of hire. *Coaching* is a day-to-day process that helps employees improve their performance. This important tool for the nurse leader encompasses many skills that can be formal or informal in nature. Some of the general behaviors of a coach include completing employee needs analysis, interviewing, decision-making, problem-solving, thinking analytically, and active listening. Once a coach has assessed his or her team, the coach can work at various strategies to motivate, mentor, and develop using communication skills.

Mentoring is a strategy that helps improve retention. *Mentoring* is a process by which a more experienced staff member guides, supports, and nurtures a less experienced person. Mentors take a greater role in staff development than preceptors.

Precepting and *preceptors* are the guides that transition new nurses (or changing practice specialties) into the clinical environment. Preceptors base their actions on professional practice standards, theory, and their patient care delivery experiences and help new nurses understand the clinical application of the knowledge they have obtained in their educational programs. Working with new nurses, preceptors are key to helping new nurses embrace and become effective patient care deliverers in a variety of clinical settings.

Performance Appraisals and Future Planning Interviews

Performance appraisals and future planning interviews are tools to not only assess an employee's performance, but also serve as an action plan or blueprint for continued development. Objective performance appraisals determine job competence, reflecting the job performance requirements. Performance appraisals are a resource to enhance staff development, determine training and developmental needs, and serve as a guideline for performance improvement. As a multifaceted tool, a performance appraisal also can assist in the communication of an employee's aspirations and provide a platform to recognize accomplishments. Although the performance appraisal can serve to identify unsatisfactory employees, this tool is not the best method to identify performance or behavior issues on an annual basis. It is best used to identify performance over a set period of time and provide a blueprint for employee development in the future.

MANAGEMENT-LABOR RELATIONSHIPS: COLLECTIVE BARGAINING

Labor-Management Relations

Across the history of business and commerce, two groups tend to form and have divergent and often conflicting interests. Different strategies may be employed to resolve conflicts between the two groups, and collective bargaining is one of them. There is a long history of dialogue in nursing about the appropriateness of nurses engaging in collective bargaining. The questions have been: Is it beneath professionalism that the nursing profession should exhibit or is collective bargaining an issue of power and autonomy to attempt to control the workplace?

The American Nurses Association (ANA) supports the rights of registered nurses to have the freedom of choice regarding their work environments and recognizes that collective bargaining is not the preferred route for some registered nurses, but is for many others. The ANA seeks to keep the interests of both nurses and patients in balance while ensuring safe and just nurse compensation and working conditions (ANA, 2012).

Decisions affecting nurses and collective bargaining have been handed down from both the National Labor Relations Board and Supreme Court. Generally, the decisions reached affect inclusion or exclusion of nurses from collective bargaining process or units and are generally based on the determination of nurses' roles as supervisors or non-supervisors in their work.

Collective Bargaining

Collective bargaining is defined as an agreement negotiated between a labor union and an employer that sets forth the terms of employment for the employees who are members of the labor union. The agreement may include provisions that pertain to wages, vacation time, working hours and conditions, and health insurance benefits. The term *collective* acknowledges that the agreements negotiated cover a defined population within an organization and are not individualized to each person.

Collective bargaining was once thought anathema to nursing and other disciplines that define themselves as professions. However, in 1946, the American Nurses Association established its Economic and General Welfare (EG&W) Program with the purpose of improving working conditions for nurses in the United States (Indiana State Nurses Association, 2006). However, the formation of the EG&W Program was not without controversy. State nurses associations, as constituents of ANA, replicated EG&W programs at the state level. Some questioned whether an association that speaks for the profession of nursing as a whole could also serve as a union for a segment of its membership. Nonetheless, most collective bargaining agreements covering registered nurses in the United States are negotiated through the labor arm of the ANA-affiliated state nurses associations.

California and Massachusetts are notable exceptions and may signal a trend toward total separation of the state organizations that represent nurses. The Massachusetts and California Nurses Associations are no longer affiliates of ANA but are part of the National Nurses United. In the wake of the schism that caused a break in the traditional organizational structure, two distinct entities now exist in each of these states—the California Nurses Association and the ANA/California in the Golden State and the Massachusetts Nurses Association and the Massachusetts Association of Registered Nurses in the Bay State.

National Nurses United is currently the largest union of registered nurses in the United States. Founded in 2009 by the unification of the Massachusetts and California Nurses Associations and the United American Nurses, this union consists of more than 185,000 members and continues to organize nurses in every state. Their mission is to advance the interests of direct care nurses, organize all direct care nurses into a single organization, promote economic and professional interests of all RNs, and promote a unified vision of collective bargaining for nurses (National Nurses United, 2012).

Negotiations

Negotiating is the mutual obligation of management and the union to meet at reasonable times and bargain in a good faith effort to reach agreement with respect to conditions of employment affecting employees represented by the union. *Conditions of employment* is a broad term that encompasses personnel policies, practices, and matters affecting working conditions. Certain matters (e.g., race, religion, gender, national origin, disability, age) are specifically excluded by law from being considered a condition of employment.

National Labor Relations Act

The National Labor Relations Act (NLRA; 29 U.S.C. Sec. 151-169, 49 Stat. 449), also known as the Wagner Act, was enacted in 1935 and is the primary law governing relations between unions and employers in the private sector. The law protects workers from the effects of unfair labor practices by employers and requires them to recognize and bargain collectively with a union that the workers elect to represent them. The NLRA guarantees employees "the right to self-organization; to form, join, or assist labor organizations; to bargain collectively through representatives of their own choosing; and to engage in concerted activities for the purpose of collective bargaining or other mutual aid and protection."

The law was enacted in the wake of widespread strikes and factory takeovers in 1933 and 1934. Violent confrontations occurred between workers trying to form unions and the police and private security forces defending the interests of anti-union employers. Some historians believe that Congress adopted the NLRA primarily in the hopes of averting even greater labor unrest. By 1945, union membership in the United States reached 35% of the workforce. In response, opponents of organized labor sought to weaken the NLRA. With the passage of the Labor–Management Relations Act (also known as Taft–Hartley) in 1947, provisions were added to the NLRA that allowed unions to be prosecuted, enjoined, and sued for a variety of activities, including mass picketing and secondary boycotts.

The National Labor Relations Board (NLRB) is an independent federal agency created by Congress to administer the NLRA. Through the years, Congress has amended the act, and the NLRB and courts have developed a body of law drawn from the statute. The last major revision of the NLRA occurred when Congress imposed further restrictions on unions through the Labor–Management Reporting and Disclosure Act of 1959 (also know as Landrum–Griffin; P.L. 86-259).

Landrum–Griffin resulted from hearings of the Senate committee on improper activities in the fields of labor and management, which uncovered evidence of collusion between dishonest employers and union officials, the use of violence by certain segments of labor leadership, and the diversion and misuse of labor union funds by high-ranking officials. The act grants certain rights to union members and protects their interests by promoting democratic procedures within labor organizations. Union members are protected against abuses by a bill of rights that includes guarantees of freedom of speech and periodic secret elections. Secondary boycotting and organizational and recognition picketing are severely restricted by the act.

Before 1974, and the amendment to the Wagner Act, it was difficult to discuss labor–management relations laws in the health services field, especially in the nonprofit sector. All facilities, both proprietary and nonprofit, became subject to the NLRA in the late 1950s by virtue of a decision of the NLRB. However, in some states, such as California, most nonprofit facilities were not subject to labor organization attempts until after the passage of the Taft–Hartley "hospital exemption." Since then, all health service institutions are now subject to the FLRA.

The importance of the 1974 Wagner Act amendment lies in the protection of patients. The amendment requires that unions must give the facility a 10-day written notice of the intent to strike prior to the strike. This allows healthcare organizations to prepare for normal operations in delivering patient care during the strike.

While nonunion facilities may not be concerned on a day-to-day basis with the NLRA, facilities with organized unions must carefully attend to the act's provisions relative to unfair labor practices, boycotts, picketing, and so forth.

Grievance and Arbitration

The negotiated grievance procedure is a system for resolving disputes. It is a method, established by the union and management, for determining where problems exist and solving those problems fairly and quickly. Every collective bargaining agreement must contain a negotiated grievance procedure.

A *grievance* is defined in the collective bargaining agreement and may cover any complaint:

- By any employee concerning any matter relating to the employment of the employee;
- By any labor organization concerning any matter relating to the employment of any employee; or
- By any employee, labor organization, or agency concerning the effect or interpretation or a claim of breach of a collective bargaining agreement or of any claimed violation, misinterpretation, or misapplication of any law, rule, or regulation affecting conditions of employment (Fair Labor Standards Act of Amendments of 1989, P.L. 101-157, 101 Stat. 1060).

Under negotiated grievance procedures, unions have the right to present and process employee or union grievances. Employees are allowed to present their own grievances (i.e., to represent themselves in the procedure) if they so desire. However, where this happens, the union has the right to be present during the process. Any negotiated grievance not satisfactorily resolved by the grievance process is subject to binding arbitration. Only the union or management may invoke arbitration.

Arbitration is a process in which an impartial third party, the *arbitrator,* is chosen by the union and management to render a final and binding award after hearing and reviewing the evidence. Because arbitration can be costly and time-consuming and can have unpredictable results, the parties to the dispute should take all necessary steps to attempt to resolve the dispute prior to calling on the arbitrator.

The union or management may file an exception to an arbitrator's award with the Federal Labor Relations Authority. This authority reviews the award to determine whether it is improper because it violates law, rule, or regulation or on other grounds similar to those applied by federal courts in private-sector labor–management relations (e.g., the arbitrator exceeded his or her authority).

The union or management has 30 days beginning on the date of an award to file exceptions with the authority. If no exceptions are filed within that time frame, then the award becomes final and binding. The refusal of either party to adhere to the award is considered an unfair labor practice.

Leading in the 21st Century

The challenge of power and autonomy in the workplace requires that nurse leaders create a culture of communication, support a constructive and productive work environment, and listen and respond to employees concerns. Nurse leaders are charged with ensuring that management's rights and employees' rights are protected. Behaviors that support an efficient and effective work environment include being aware of early signs of employee discontent, structuring the environment to support empowerment and autonomy, and advocating for nurses values and needs.

The movement toward collective bargaining interdisciplinary teams and the movement toward collective bargaining in nursing are in conflict and are ethical issues for nurses. Nurse leaders are challenged to strike a balance among competing needs and values and to create and maintain a positive work climate and high-quality client outcomes. Unionization versus professionalism is a power and autonomy issue in nursing that leaders and managers need to deal with in the work environment.

HEALTHCARE POLICY AND POLITICS

Nursing has a strong legacy of political activism affecting public health policy. The delivery of nursing care is affected by social and healthcare policies. Nurse leaders are charged with developing influence in the four connected spheres of influence to support nursing as a discipline with a general goal to improve the health of people.

The workplace is a sphere where policies and procedures define a nurse's work setting. Examples of policies and procedure include overtime regulations, designated smoking areas, and staffing ratios. Magnet facilities attempt to offer shared governance models and nurse-driven policies in the workplace.

Professional organizations are another sphere of political influence that are instrumental in shaping the practice of nursing. Organizations can be a significant force in the development of broader health and social policies to address social issues. Nursing organizations need to work together to advocate for patients, nursing, and health care at the clinical practice and national levels.

The community is a sphere of influence and can include a neighborhood or it can be an international online group with a common interest. Nurses are members of communities and have a responsibility to promote the welfare of the community and its members.

The government is a sphere of influence that requires nurse leaders to be actively involved because government plays an enormous role in nursing and health care. Actions of the government touch every part of our lives as evidenced in the examples of laws and regulations such as childhood immunizations, legal drinking alcohol age, and voting.

Healthcare policy is established largely through government agencies, chief among them the U.S. Department of Health and Human Services at the national level and department equivalents at the state level. One of the most recent health policy issues in the United States in healthcare reform is the Patient Access and Affordability Care Act.

Nurses need to embrace healthy policy at a grassroots level where they can make a difference in the outcome of policies being accepted or rejected. Some nurses will advance further in health policy by running for office or accepting political appointments such as state commissioner of health.

It is incumbent upon nurses to understand how policy develops in the form of legislation. Nurses need to know how a bill becomes law at both the federal and state levels (see Figure 6–1).

FIGURE 6–1.
EXAMPLE OF A STATE'S PROCESS FOR A BILL BECOMING A LAW

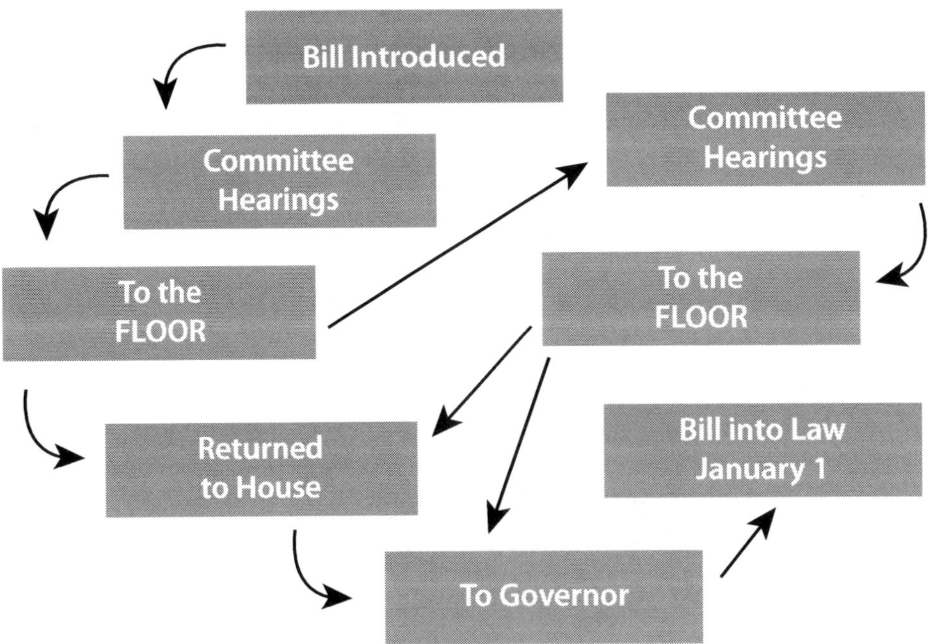

Making a difference in healthcare policy requires being involved. Steps to being involved include becoming an active participant in the form of a grassroots advocate, for example, taking the initiative to write letters to the editor of publications about issues about which nurses are passionate. Another responsibility and method to have nursing's voice heard is to call, write, and email legislative officials about issues and pending legislation. A simple path to knowledge regarding those issues can be by routinely accessing the Library of Congress at http://thomas.loc.gov. Routinely viewing the ANA's Government Affairs webpage provides updates, alerts, and information that support being an active participant in the healthcare policy process, including ANA's legislative agenda for each Congress. Lastly, being involved might include facilitating a voter registration campaign to encourage and educate nurses about the importance of having a voice in the direction of healthcare policy at the local, state, regional, or national level.

The following initiatives are among the most significant for the development of broad-based health policy in the current and coming decades.

- ***Healthy People: Understanding and Improving Health.*** Published under the auspices of the U.S. Public Health Service, this text builds on the seminal document first issued in 1991 and on *Healthy People 2000: National Health Promotion and Disease Prevention Objectives*. National healthcare initiatives continue in the form of *Healthy People 2020* .

  Healthy People 2020 serves as the prevention agenda for the United States. It is a statement of national health objectives designed to identify the most significant preventable threats to health and to establish national goals to reduce these threats.

  Healthy People is managed by the Office of Disease Prevention and Health Promotion, U.S. Department of Health and Human Services. It has two main goals: The first is to help individuals of all ages increase life expectancy and improve their quality of life, and the second is to eliminate health disparities among different segments of the population.

- ***Guidelines of the U.S. Public Health Service's Centers for Disease Control and Prevention.***
  The recommended prevention guidelines, designed to keep people healthy, are used as a reference point for health promotion by a multitude of health plans throughout the United States.

- ***Clinical Practice Guidelines for the U.S. Public Health Service's AHRQ.*** Numerous evidence-based guidelines for practice, written from both the client's and the provider's perspectives, are available through AHRQ (see http://www.ahcpr.gov/).

Goals for future healthcare policy continue to be a need to focus on the quality of health care through prevention and consumer health literacy as well as accessibility to health care. Another goal that needs continued attention includes the financial strength and sustainability of Medicare and other programs to fund healthcare delivery and services provided. Nursing's involvement in the political process is a responsibility and competency that has an ongoing impact on the health of patients, families, communities, and populations.

ETHICS

Professional Ethics

Professions are defined, in part, by the ethics that govern their practice. While nursing has long been recognized for its commitment to high ethical standards, that commitment was further endorsed in 1990 with the establishment of the Center for Ethics and Human Rights under the aegis of the ANA. The center is "committed to addressing the complex ethical and human rights issues confronting nurses and designing activities and programs to increase the ethical competence and human rights sensitivity of nurses" (ANA, 2009). The rich library of resources available through the center is found at http://www.nursingworld.org/ethics (Bobinski, Hall, & Orentlicher, 2007).

Values Clarification and Cultural Diversity

The diverse beliefs and value systems that clients/patients, staff, and practitioners bring with them to the healthcare environment speak to the need for managers to expand their knowledge of diversity from an ethical as well as from a business perspective.

Dimensions of diversity include age, gender, sexual orientation, ability/disability, ethnicity, socioeconomic status, education, origin, and so forth. The Code of Ethics that governs the practice of nursing compels managers to practice "with compassion and respect for the inherent dignity, worth, and uniqueness of every individual, unrestricted by considerations of social or economic status, personal attributes, or the nature of health problems" (ANA, 2001, p. 4).

The healthcare executive is challenged to integrate and interpret disparate points of view among and within the staff he or she manages as well as among and between the client groups served and the staff who serve them. For example, there may be no words in "high-context" languages to compare with the "low-context" English terminology used to explain certain procedures or interventions. Imagine attempting to explain "do not resuscitate" to someone who has no reference point for the concept of *resuscitation.*

Professional Integrity

Integrity is defined as strict adherence to a code of conduct that is above reproach. The hallmarks of a profession are noted as

- Extended education (body of knowledge) that sets its members apart;
- Theoretical body of knowledge leading to defined skills, abilities, and norms;
- Provision of a specific practice (of value to society and for which society cannot provide independent of the profession);
- Autonomy in decision-making and practice;
- Existence of a code of ethics that governs the practice of the members of the profession.

Managers have an ongoing opportunity to exemplify professional integrity in their work and to influence the practice of their subordinates by example.

Code for Nurses

The abbreviated version of the Code of Ethics for Nurses is presented in Box 6–1. The full *Code for Nurses With Interpretive Statements* monograph (ANA, 2001) is available through ANA. Further information about obtaining the booklet can be found at http://www.nursingworld.org/codeofethics.

BOX 6–1.
CODE OF ETHICS FOR NURSES

1. The nurse, in all professional relationships, practices with compassion and respect for the inherent dignity, worth, and uniqueness of every individual, unrestricted by considerations of social or economic status, personal attributes, or the nature of health problems.
2. The nurse's primary commitment is to the patient, whether an individual, family group, or community.
3. The nurse promotes, advocates for, and strives to protect the health, safety, and rights of the patient.
4. The nurse is responsible and accountable for individual nursing practice and determines the appropriate delegation of tasks consistent with the nurse's obligation to provide optimum patient care.
5. The nurse owes the same duties to self as to others, including the responsibility to preserve integrity and safety, to maintain competence, and to continue personal and professional growth.
6. The nurse participates in establishing, maintaining, and improving healthcare environments and conditions of employment conducive to the provision of quality health care and consistent with the values of the profession through individual and collective action.
7. The nurse participates in the advancement of the profession through contributions to practice, education, administration, and knowledge development.
8. The nurse collaborates with other health professionals and the public in promoting community, national, and international efforts to meet health needs.
9. The profession of nursing, as represented by associations and their members, is responsible for articulating nursing values, for maintaining the integrity of the profession and its practice, and for shaping social policy.

Reprinted from *Code of ethics for nurses with interpretive statements* (p. 4) by the American Nurses Association, 2001, Silver Spring, MD: Author.

Confidentiality

The absolute need to maintain confidentiality in practice is a tenet so dear that its violation may, under certain circumstances, result in immediate termination of employment. With the implementation of HIPAA, civil and criminal penalties can be levied when legal requirements regarding confidentiality are ignored or violated.

Refusal of Assignment

Staff members retain the right to refuse an assignment based on their own deeply held beliefs. This situation usually arises in cases involving termination of pregnancy or withdrawal of life support. In the coming years, managers and administrators should anticipate the potential dilemmas related to genetic engineering and its possible impact on the acceptance or refusal of assignments by staff members.

Ethical Theories

Two major theoretical perspectives form the foundation for dialogue about ethical issues pertinent to health care: (1) the deontological approach and (2) the teleological approach. *Deontology* holds that an act is good unto itself. It is sometimes described as the theory rooted in "rules," as it holds that certain rules must be followed or actions taken regardless of the consequences. For example, if the belief is that the truth must always be told, there is no reason to not tell the truth, under any circumstance.

On the other hand, theorists in *teleology* hold that the end or purpose of an action determines its rightness or wrongness. Utilitarianism is the prime example of the teleological belief system. Utility holds that "the greatest good for the greatest number" is the desired end point and that the relative "right" or "wrong" of acts is less important that the consequence of those acts. For example, it may be morally acceptable for a mother to steal a loaf of bread to feed her family if the only other option open to her is their starvation.

Ethical Principles

Here, briefly described, are the major ethical principles that guide those in the field of health care:

- *Respect for persons.* Human beings are *autonomous,* that is, they have the capacity for rational action and moral choice and have a value unto themselves. Their choices and judgment should be respected and should not be interfered with unless they are clearly harmful to others. The degree of autonomy varies to some degree according to the person's capacity for decision-making and choice on his or her own behalf. For example, the infant has the potential for autonomy but not yet the capacity. In addition to autonomy, *veracity* (truth-telling), *confidentiality*, and *informed consent* are derived from the principle of respect for persons.

- *Beneficence,* which holds that first, one has an obligation to do no harm, and second, one has an obligation to promote good. The principle of beneficence is basic to medicine. The extent to which beneficence and autonomy are competing values rests at the heart of discourse about ethical dilemmas (see below). For example, if the physician believes that, with another round of aggressive radiation, she may "buy more time" for the patient, but the patient, who is aware and fully informed, chooses to forgo the radiation with the knowledge that his decision will certainly hasten death, then the patient's desire for autonomy and the physician's commitment to beneficence may be in conflict.
- *Justice,* which as an ethical principle means "that which is fair or that which is deserved." The concept of *rights* is associated with justice, as is the notion of *obligation.* The ethical issues surrounding allocation of resources often are seen as promoting or neglecting the principle of justice. For example, a patient with a predictably terminal illness hears about a costly experimental treatment for his disease, wants to have the treatment, and asks his health maintenance organization (HMO) to assume the cost of the treatment. The HMO refuses because the action would be precedent setting and the principle of justice held by the organization—the "most good for the most people"—would be vaulted. Utilitarian justice guides the decision in this case (Lachman, 2005).

Ethical Dilemmas

An *ethical dilemma* exists in the presence of competing values in which the community, as well as the individuals involved, has a vested interest. Healthcare institutions have formalized the existence of multidisciplinary ethics committees as advisory bodies to help sort through the dilemmas faced by patients, their caregivers, and their families.

A systematic approach to the identification and meaning of the ethical issues is suggested. One such approach is outlined by those involved in the Ethics in Medicine Division of the University of Washington's School of Medicine. The recommended "ethics work-up" includes a review of medical indications, patient preferences, quality of life, and contextual issues. The work-up describes "what is." Then, the deliberation moves to the next phase and involves questions such as these:

- What is at issue?
- Where is the conflict?
- What is this case about? Is it similar to other cases encountered? What is known about them?
- Is there precedent? Is there a paradigm case (e.g., Karen Ann Quinlan, Nancy Cruzan, and Terri Schiavo [see p. 148])?
- Who is involved, and what roles do they play?

Another model to address ethical issues is the following:

- Identify the problem.
- Tease out the ethical problem/dilemma.
- Gather objective and subjective data.
- Look at alternatives.
- Study the consequences of the alternatives.
- Select the most appropriate alternative.
- Compare the selected alternative with the clinician's/executive's value system.

Cultural values may be at the center of ethical dilemmas. For example, the commitment to honor end-of-life care preferences has been codified, and patients are now routinely asked about the availability of an advance directive for health care or a living will. If the patient's background is such that death is a taboo subject, perhaps because of a belief system that holds that to speak of death invites him in the door, then discussions about life support or the withdrawal of life supporting interventions may be inappropriate from the standpoint of the family and patient but is greatly desired by the healthcare team.

Ethics and Human Values

Patient/Client Rights

The concept of patient/client rights has taken on new importance in recent years. In 1973, the American Hospital Association published a list of patient rights that has been used as issued or in slightly edited versions since that time. (Each state also publishes its own list of patient rights.) Patients are generally provided with a copy of their rights upon entry into the acute care setting; similar rights are accorded those in LTC, rehabilitation care, and so forth. State law may mandate such provisions. A patient's rights include

- The right to considerate and respectful care.
- The right to receive complete, up-to-date information about diagnosis, treatment, and prognosis (expected outcome) from his or her physician in terms the patient can reasonably be expected to understand. If it is not medically advisable to give this information to the patient, it should be given to another appropriate person on his or her behalf. The patient (or the appropriate person) has the right to know by name the physician who is responsible for coordinating the care of the patient.
- The right to receive enough information about any proposed treatment or procedure to make an *informed consent*—that is, he or she should know enough about the expected benefits, possible hazards, and time needed for recovery to decide if he or she wants that treatment or procedure. This information should come from the patient's doctor and should be provided in every case except those emergencies in which a delay could harm the patient.

- The right to be told about alternatives to the proposed treatment or procedure and the right to know who will be responsible for the treatment or procedure.
- The right to refuse treatment to the extent permitted by law and to be informed of the possible medical consequences of doing so.
- The right to every consideration of privacy concerning his or her own medical care program. Case discussion, consultation, examination, and treatment are confidential and should be conducted discreetly. Those not directly involved in his or her care must have the permission of the patient to be present.
- The right to expect that all communications and records concerning his or her care should be treated as confidential.
- The right to expect the hospital to make a reasonable response to his or her request for services. Depending on how urgent the patient's medical problem, the hospital must evaluate the patient and then must provide service or referral. If the patient is to be transferred to another facility, he or she must first receive all the information and an explanation of why a transfer must be made. The institution to which the patient is to be transferred must accept the patient before he or she is transferred. The patient has the right to be informed of any relationships the hospital has to any other health care or education institutions if the relationship may affect his or her care.
- The right to know if any of the people treating him or her have any professional relationships among themselves that might affect his or her care.
- The right to be told if the hospital plans to engage in any human experimentation that might affect his or her care or treatment. The patient has the right to refuse to participate in such research projects.
- The right to expect reasonable continuity of care. He or she has the right to know in advance what appointment times and physicians are available and where they will be. The patient has the right to be informed about what his or her continuing healthcare requirements will be after discharge.
- The right to examine and receive an explanation of his or her bill regardless of whether it's paid by him or her or another source.
- The right to know what hospital rules and regulations apply to his or her conduct as a patient.

Advocacy

Advocates are those who stand in for or plead the cause of those who cannot speak for themselves. Nurses often described themselves as "patient advocates." However, because nurses are accountable to constituencies whose values are occasionally at odds with one another, the assumption that the nurse will always act as a patient advocate may present an ethical dilemma. When faced with such a quandry, nurses may elect to apply an ethical framework as part of their decision-making process. Here is one approach:

- What are the medical/healthcare issues present in the situation?
- What are the patient's preferences (to the extent they are known or can be discovered)?
- What is the quality of life for the patient (from his or her perspective, not that of the nurse)?
- What is the context surrounding the situation? What familial, legal, economic, or institutional matters must be considered as part of the deliberations? (Sugarman & Sulmasy, 2001)

Advance Directives

The Patient Self Determination Act of 1990 (PSDA) requires that all individuals receiving medical care must be given written information about their rights under state law to make decisions about their care, including the right to accept or refuse medical or surgical treatment. Individuals also must be given information about their rights to formulate advance directives such as living wills and durable powers of attorney for health care. Patients must be made aware of their rights to make decisions about these issues upon admission (in the case of hospitals or skilled nursing facilities), enrollment (in the case of HMOs), on first receipt of care (in the case of hospices), or before the patient comes under an agency's care (in the case of home health–personal care agencies).

Nurses have a critical role to play in end-of-life care, and the voice of the profession is very much in evidence because of initiatives such as the End-of Life Nursing Education Consortium (ELNEC) project. In collaboration with the Robert Wood Johnson Foundation, the American Association of Colleges of Nursing began the ELNEC project in 2000. ELNEC is a national education initiative to improve end-of-life care in the United States. The project provides nurse educators with training in end-of-life care so they can teach this essential information to nursing students and practicing nurses (Matzo, Sherman, Penn, & Ferrell, 2003).

Organ Donation and Transplants

The number of people on waiting lists for organ transplants far exceeds available organs. For the most part, those whose names are at the top of most lists are people who have become so seriously ill that they need to receive viable organs within a relatively short time to forestall inevitable death. To ensure equity in the distribution of scarce organs, a computer databank has been established. Its intent is to quickly match donors with recipients and to facilitate the delivery of organs in a timely manner to increase the probability of successful transplantation (Sheehy et al., 2003).

A few of the topical ethical issues surrounding organ donation include the following:

- Do people have the "right" to bypass the organ donor system and petition for organs via the Internet?
- If the person is successful in procuring an organ, is the healthcare system under any obligation to perform the transplant?

- Is it acceptable to "purchase" organs or to offer some type of financial recompense for donated organs?
- Should "healthier" transplant candidates be placed at the top of the waiting list in preference to those who are very ill so that the donated organs will "last longer"?
- Do uninsured poor individuals have the same right to organs as those with insurance? If the answer is yes, who assumes financial risk for the procedure and for follow-up care?
- Do people wanting experimental transplant procedures have the right to expect their managed care insurer to pay for the procedure contrary to the terms of the agreement with the carrier?
- Rather than requesting permission to proceed with organ removal in the face of an inevitable outcome of death, should the medical community assume consent and automatically harvest much-needed organs?

Soon, ethical dilemmas related to genetics, including DNA manipulation and organ cloning, will overshadow the ethical quandaries posed by organ donation and transplantation.

Resource Utilization

Ethical concerns surround the allocation of scarce resources in the field of health care. Perhaps the most cogent question is the one that is seldom asked: If waste were to be removed from the system, would resources still be scarce? While ethicists and philosophers debate the question around the theme of justice, those on the frontline of the delivery system make daily decisions that compel them to say "no" to some objective good so that they can say "yes" to a competing need (Lachman, 2009).

At least one healthcare system in the United States has taken ethical discourse beyond that which ponders case-by-case dilemmas at the bedside and brought the discussion into the boardroom where top-level decision-makers have agreed to add an ethical filter to their resource allocation deliberations (Cavalier & Ess, n.d.). The degree to which this approach will be adopted more widely is unknown at this time.

Business Ethics

Ethical challenges present themselves not only in clinical practice, but also in the practice of organizational operations. *Business ethics* is defined as the critical, structured examination of how people and institutions should behave in the world of commerce. It involves examining appropriate constraints on the pursuit of self-interest, or (for firms) profits, when the actions of individuals or firms affects others (Business Ethics.ca, 2012). Business ethics impact healthcare organizations in light of the challenges where the dollar amount spent to provide services grows daily, and the pace of change in delivering care is accelerating almost daily. How to keep healthcare organizations legal, ethical, and funded is the ongoing challenge that can and does produce ethical conflict for nurse leaders in an environment where business ethics and patient care ethics often seem to be at odds.

Clinical ethics and organizational ethics often are in conflict secondary to diminishing resources. Nurse executives remain committed to the organization, the nursing staff and profession, and their own value system. Often nurse executives must strike a balance among these factors.

Landmark Ethical Cases

Karen Ann Quinlan: Karen Ann was in a persistent vegetative state and was ventilator-dependent in the 1970s. Her parents determined that she would not want to live the rest of her life in this manner. Because life support had never been discontinued, an attorney in New Jersey took the Quinlans' case to the New Jersey Supreme Court. The court ruled that the ventilator could be discontinued. The decision was based on the Constitution of the United States and the right to privacy. The court decision permitted surrogate decision-making and, in New Jersey, advised that every hospital should establish a bioethics committee because such cases could best be handled by medical professionals and not the courts.

Nancy Ellen Jobes: Nancy Ellen had been involved in a motor vehicle accident. She required surgery and sustained brain damage as a result of the anesthesia. She was in a persistent vegetative state on tube-feeding for 6 years. Her husband and her parents determined that she would not want to live the rest of her life in this manner. The same attorney in New Jersey that handled the Quinlan case decided to assist the family of Nancy Ellen. This case also went to the New Jersey Supreme Court. The question that the court had to consider was the following: Can artificial tube-feeding be discontinued, or is this an essential component of life? Based on case precedence from the Quinlan decision, the New Jersey State Supreme Court ruled that the artificial tube-feeding could be discontinued.

Nancy Beth Cruzan: Nancy Beth was resuscitated at the scene of a motor vehicle accident in which she was involved. Like Nancy Ellen Jobes, she was in a persistent vegetative state being maintained on artificial tube-feeding for several years in a Missouri rehabilitation hospital. Her parents determined that she would not want to live the rest of her life in this manner. Her case went to the Missouri State Supreme Court. Unlike Quinlan and Jobes, the Missouri State Supreme Court denied the request to have the artificial tube-feeding discontinued. The court based their decision on a lack of evidence to support that Nancy Beth would not want to live in this manner. The Cruzans' attorney petitioned the United States Supreme Court to hear the case. The U.S. Supreme Court heard the case, but did not make a decision. They stated that it was up to each state to handle such cases; however, they recommended that if every patient had an advanced directive, such a directive would serve as evidence of how the patient would want to live if such circumstances existed. The Patient Self Determination Act of 1990 is a direct result of the Cruzan court decision.

The Cruzans had to go again before the Missouri State Supreme Court. This time, individuals such as family and friends demonstrated how Nancy Beth would not want to live in this manner. They showed the court videos of how active she was and how she enjoyed life. The Missouri State Supreme Court ruled to have to the artificial tube-feeding discontinued. Following the artificial tube-feeding removal, Nancy Beth Cruzan died on December 26, 1990. Nancy Beth's tombstone bears three significant dates representative of the family's plight to have the tube-feeding removed.

Terri Ann Schiavo: The Schiavo case probably best ties together law, ethics, and morals. Terri Ann Schiavo had an eating disorder and most likely suffered cardiac arrest from an electrolyte abnormality. She was resuscitated and was maintained on artificial tube-feeding in a persistent vegetative state for many years. Her husband determined that she would not want to live in this manner. Her parents wanted everything done for her because they felt that her condition was improving. A renowned neurologist determined that Terri Ann was in a persistent vegetative state. The case made its way to the Florida State Supreme Court. This court ruled that the artificial tube-feeding could be discontinued. Terri Ann's parents requested the U.S. Supreme Court hear this case, but the court refused to do so, making the Florida State Supreme Court decision final. The tube-feeding was removed and Terri Ann died.

This case ties law, ethics, and morals together. Terri Ann's husband was the legal decision-maker because he was still her legal spouse. This case also represents how conflicts between family members create ethical dilemmas. It is interesting to note that the husband of Terri Ann Schiavo is a nurse. Terri Ann's body was moved to Pennsylvania, where she was laid to rest.

REFERENCES

About.com-Economics. (2009). *Definition of human capital.* Retrieved from http://economics.about.com/cs/economicsglossary/g/human_capital.htm

Aid to Families with Dependent Children, P.L. 74-271, 49 Stat. 620.

Age Discrimination in Employment Act of 1967, P.L. 90-202, 81 Stat. 602.

Agency for Healthcare Research and Quality. (n.d.). *Making health safer: A critical analysis of patient safety practices.* Available online at http://www.ahcpr.gov/clinic/ptsafety/

American Nurses Association. (2012). *Union facts.* Retrieved from http://www.unionfacts.com/union/american_nurses_association

American Nurses Association. (2001). *Code of ethics for nurses with interpretive statements.* Washinton, DC: Author.

American Nurses Association. (2009). *Nursing ethics.* Retrieved from http://www.nursingworld.org/MainMenuCategories/EthicsStandards.aspx

American Nurses Association. (2012). *Health & safety: Collective bargaining.* Retrieved from http://www.nursingworld.org/MainMenuCategories/WorkplaceSafety/Work-Environment/Collective-Bargaining

American Recovery and Reinvestment Act of 2009, P.L. 111-5.

Americans with Disabilities. (2012). *ADA.* Retrieved from http://www.ada.gov/pubs/ada.htm

Balanced Budget Act of 1997, P.L. 105-33, 111 Stat. 251.

Bateman, T., & Snell, S. (2002). *Management: Competing in the new era* (5th ed.). Boston: McGraw-Hill/Irwin.

Beauchamp, T. L., Bowie, N. E., & Arnold, D. G. (Eds.). (2008). *Ethical theory and business* (8th ed.). Upper Saddle River, NJ: Prentice Hall, Inc.

Beecroft, P. C., Kunzman, L., & Krozek, C. (2001). RN internship: Outcomes of a one-year pilot program. *Journal of Nursing Administration, 31*(12), 575–582.

Bennis, W., & Thomas, R. (2002, September). Crucibles of leadership. *Harvard Business Review, 80*(9), 39–45.

Benner, P. (1984). *From novice to expert: Excellence and power in clinical nursing practice.* Menlo Park, CA: Addison-Wesley.

Benner, P., Tanner, C., & Chesla, C. (1996). *Expertise in nursing practice: Caring, clinical judgment, and ethics.* New York: Springer.

Bobinski, M. A., Hall, M. A., & Orentlicher, D. (2007). *Health care law and ethics* (7th ed.). New York: Wolters Kluwer/Aspen.

Brown, D. W. (2009). The dawn of Healthy People 2020: A brief look at its beginnings. *Preventive Medicine, 48*(1), 94–95.

Budd, K. W., Warino, L. S., & Patton, M. E. (2004). Traditional and non-traditional collective bargaining: Strategies to improve the patient care environment. *Online Journal of Issues in Nursing.* Retrieved from http://www.ncbi.nlm.nih.gov/pubmed/14998358

Buerhaus, P. I., Donelan, K., Ulrich, B.T., Norman, L., & Dittus, R. (2006). State of registered nurses workforce in the United States. *Nursing Economics, 24*(1), 6–12.

Bureau of Labor Statistics. (2012). *Wagner Act.* Retrieved from http://www.bls.gov/opub/rtaw/pdf/lrtime.pdf

Cavalier, R., & Ess, C. (ND). *Introduction to Habermas's discourse ethics.* Retrieved from http://caae.phil.cmu.edu/Cavalier/Forum/meta/background/HaberIntro.html

Centers for Disease Control and Prevention. (2009). *Summary Health Statistics for U.S. Adults: National Health Interview Survey, 2009.* Retrieved from http://www.cdc.gov/nchs/data/series/sr_10/sr10_249.pdf

Centers for Disease Control and Prevention . (2010). *Summary Health Statistics for the U.S. Population: National Health Interview. Survey, 2009.* Series 10, Number 248. Retrieved from www.cdc.gov/nchs/data/series/sr_10/sr10_248.pdf

Centers for Disease Control and Prevention. (2011a). *National Center for Health Statistics.* Retrieved from http://www.cdc.gov/nchs/index.htm

Centers for Disease Control and Prevention. (2011b). *National Center for Health Statistics, FastStats.* Retrieved from http://www.cdc.gov/nchs/fastats/default.htm

Center for Generational Studies. (2009-2012). Retrieved from http://www.generationaldiversity.com/index.php

Centers for Medicare & Medicaid Services. (2005). *Overview: Medicare program general information.* Retrieved from http://www.cms.hhs.gov/MedicareGenInfo/

Children's Health Insurance Act Reauthorization Act of 2009, P.L. 111-03, 123 Stat. 30.

Civil Rights Act of 1964, P.L. 88-352, 78 Stat. 241.

Civil Rights Act of 1991, P.L. 102-162, 105 Stat. 1071.

Civil Service Reform Act of 1978, P.L. 95-454, 92 Stat. 1111.

Connor, D. (1995). *Managing at the speed of change: How resilient managers succeed and prosper where others fail.* New York: Villard Books.

Consolidated Omnibus Budget Reconciliation Act of 1986, P.L. 99-272, 100 Stat. 82.

Consumer Credit Protection Act, P. L. 90-321; 82 Stat. 146 (1968).

Consumer Financial Protection Bureau. (2012). *About us.* Retrieved from http://www.consumerfinance.gov/the-bureau

Deming, W. E. (2000). *Out of the crisis.* Boston: MIT Press.

EEOC. (n.d.-a). *About the EEOC: Overview.* Retrieved from http://www.eeoc.gov/eeoc/index.cfm

EEOC. (n.d.-b). *EEOC: Sexual harrassment.* Retrieved from http://www.eeoc.gov/laws/types/sexual_harassment.cfm

EEOC. (n.d.-c). *Enforcement guidance: workers' compensation and the ADA.* Retrieved from http://www.eeoc.gov/docs/workcomp.html

The Employment Law Group. (2011).*The SEC's new rules for the Dodd-Frank whistleblower program.* Retrieved from http://www.employmentlawgroup.net/Articles/ROswald/TheSECsNewRulesForTheDoddFrankWhistleblowerProgram.html

Equal Pay Act of 1963, P.L. 88-38, 77 Stat. 56, 59.

Exec. Order 11246 41 C.F.R. 60.

Fair Labor Standards Act, P.L. 99-239, 99 Stat. 1770 (1938).

Fair Labor Standards Act Amendments of 1989, P.L. 101-157, 101 Stat. 1060.

Foster, N. (Ed.). (2000). *Doing what counts for patient safety: Federal actions to reduce medical errors and their impact.* Rockville, MD: Quality Interagency Coordination Task Force. Available at http://www.quic.gov/report/errors6.pdf

Garrett, T. M., Ballie, H. M., & Garrett, R. M. (2009). *Health care ethics: Principles and problems* (5th ed.). Upper Saddle River, NJ: Prentice Hall.

Gingerich, B. S. (2002). National Committee for Quality Assurance. *Home Health Care Management & Practice, 14*(5), 387–388.

Greenwald, H., & Beery, W. (2002). *Health for all: Making community collaboration work.* Chicago: Health Administration Press.

Griffith, J., & White, K. (2002). *The well-managed healthcare organization* (5th ed.). Chicago: Health Administration Press

Grol, R., Berwick, D. M., & Wensing, M. (2008). On the trail of quality and safety in healthcare. *BMJ, 336,* 74–76.

Health Insurance Portability and Accountability and Accessibility Act of 1996, P.L. 104-191, 110 Stat. 1936.

Healthfield, S. M. (n.d.). *Employee satisfaction.* Retrieved from http://humanresources.about.com/od/employeesurvey1/g/employee_satisfy.htm

Healthfield, S. (2012). *Employee benefits package: What's in a comprehensive employee benefits package?* Retrieved from: http://humanresources.about.com/od/compensation-structure/tp/employee-benefits-package.htm

Henry J. Kaiser Family Foundation. (2008). *Employee health benefits: 2008 annual survey.* Menlo Park, CA: Author

Hughes, A., Sathe, N., & Spagnola, K. (2008). *State estimates of substance use from the 2005–2006 national surveys on drug use and Health* (DHHS Publication No. SMA 08-4311, NSDUH Series H-33). Rockville, MD: Substance Abuse and Mental Health Services Administration, Office of Applied Studies.

Hyde, J., & Cook, M. J. (2004). *Managing and supporting people in health care.* Oxford, UK: Baillière Tindall/Elsevier.

Immigration Act of 1990, P.L. 101-649, 104 Stat. 4978-5087.

Indiana State Nurses Association. (2006). *Economic and general welfare of nurses.* Retrieved from http://www.indiananurses.org/workplace/economic_program.htm

The Joint Commission. (2009, October 13). *Facts about The Joint Commission.* Retrieved from http://www.jointcommission.org/AboutUs/Fact_Sheets/joint_commission_facts.htm

Jones, N. (1997, July). *The electronic medical record, clinical guidelines and evidence-based medicine.* Retrieved from http://www.racgp.aone.net.au/papers/jones2.htm

Labor–Management Relations Act of 1947, 29 USCS § 141.

Labor–Management Reporting and Disclosure Act of 1959, P.L. 86-257, 73 Stat. 519-546.

Lachman, V. (2005). *Applied ethics in nursing.* New York: Springer.

Lachman, V. (2009). *Ethical challenges in healthcare: Developing your moral compass.* New York: Springer.

Mason, D. J., Leavitt, J. K., & Chaffe, M. W. (2007). *Policy & politics in nursing and health care* (5th ed.). St. Louis, MO: W.B. Saunders/Elsevier.

Matzo, M. L., Sherman, D. W., Penn, B., & Ferrell, B.R. (2003). The End-of-Life Nursing Education Consortium (ELNAC) experience. *Nurse Educator, 28*(6), 266–270.

Medicare Prescription Drug and Modernization Act of 1973, P. L. 108-173, 117 Stat. 206.

National Labor Relations Act, 29 U.S.C. Sec. Sec. 151-169, 49 Stat. 449 (1935).

National Nurses United. (2010-2012). *Home page.* Retrieved from http://www.nationalnursesunited.org/

Occupational Safety and Health Act of 1970, P.L. 91-596, 84 Stat. 1590.

Occupational Safety and Health Administration. (2005). *OSHA Directive Number CPL 02-00-137: Fatality/ catastrophe investigation procedures.* Washington, DC: Author. Available at http://www.osha.gov/ OshDoc/Directive_pdf/CPL_02-00-137.pdf

Occupational Safety and Health Administration. (2007). *Frequently asked questions: August 2007.* Retrieved from http://www.osha.gov/as/opa/osha-faq.html

Occupational Safety and Health Administration. (2008). *OSHA's role.* Retrieved from http://www.osha.gov/ oshinfo/mission.html

Occupational Safety and Health Administration. (2009). *Accident investigation search.* Retrieved from http://www.osha.gov/pls/imis /accidentsearch.html

Office of Inspector General of the U.S. Department of Health and Human Services and the American Health Lawyers Association. (n.d.). *Corporate responsibility and corporate compliance: A resource for health care boards of directors.* Retrieved from http://oig.hhs.gov/fraud/docs/complianceguidance/0402 03CorpRespRsceGuide.pdf

Patient Self-Determination Act of Omnibus Reconciliation Act of 1990, P.L. 101-508, Sections 4206 and 4751.

Personal Responsibility and Work Opportunity Reconciliation Act of 1996, P.L. 104-193, 110 Stat. 2105.

Pitman, J. (2007). Registered nurse job satisfaction and collective bargaining unit membership status. *Journal of Nursing Administration, 37*(10), 471–476.

Poe, L. (2008). Nursing regulation, the nurse licensure compact, and nurse administrators working together for patient safety. *Nursing Administration Quarterly, 32*(4), 267–272.

Pregnancy Discrimination Act, P.L. 95-555, 92 Stat. 2076 (1978).

Purnell, L. D., & Paulanka, B. J. (2008). *Transcultural health care: A culturally competent approach.* Philadelphia: F.A. Davis.

Puskin, D. (2001, September 30). Telemedicine: Follow the money. *Online Journal of Issues in Nursing.* Retrieved from http://www.nursingworld.org/ojin/topic16/tpc16_1.htm

Rehabilitation Act of 1973, P.L.93-112, 87 Stat. 394.

Rollert, J. P. (n.d.) *Six principles for business ethics.* Retrieved from http://www.huffingtonpost.com/john-paul-rollert/six-principles-for-busine_b_1660847.html

Roussel, L. (Ed.). (2013). *Management and leadership for nurse administrators.* Burlington, MA: Jones & Bartlett Learning.

Santora, J., Caro, M., & Sarros, J. (2007). Succession in nonprofit organizations: An insider/outsider perspective. *SAM Advanced Management Journal, 72*(4), 26–31. Retrieved from Business Source Complete database.

Sheehy, E., Conrad, S. L., Brigham, L. E., Luskin, R., Weber, P., Eakin, M., et al. (2003). Estimating the number of potential organ donors in the United States. *New England Journal of Medicine, 349,* 2073–2075.

Shi, L., & Singh, D. A. (2008). *Delivering health care in America: A systems approach.* Sudbury, MA: Jones & Bartlett.

Shipp, P. L., & Davison, C. J. (2001). Leveraging diversity: It takes a system. *Leadership in Action, 20*(6), 1–5. Retrieved from: http://media.wiley.com/assets/51/56/jrnls_jb_lia_shipp.pdf

Shojania, K.G., Duncan, B. W., McDonald, K. M., & Wachter, R. M. (Eds.). (2001). Making health care safer: A critical analysis of patient safety practices. *AHRQ, 43.*

Slocum, J. W. (1981). Job redesign: Improving the quality of work life. *Journal of Experiential Learning and Simulation, 3*(1), 17–36

Smith, V., Krugman, M., & Oman, K. (2005). Evaluating the impact of computerized clinical documentation. *CIN: Computers Informatics Nursing, 23*(3), 132–138.

Sugarman, J., & Sulmasy, D. P. (Eds). (2001). *Methods in medical ethics.* Washington, DC: Georgetown University Press.

Social Security Amendments of 1965, P.L. 89-97, 79 Stat. 286.

Social Security Amendments of 1972, P.L. 92-603, 86 Stat. 1329.

Spath, P. (Ed.). (2002). *Guide to effective staff development in health care organizations: A systems approach to successful training.* San Francisco: Jossey-Bass.

Stockho, A. (1999, November/December). Scenario planning: A useful tool in building strategic intent. *Health Progress.* Retrieved from http://www.chausa.org/PUBS/PUBSART.ASP?ISSUE=HP9911&ARTICLE=O

Upenieks, V. (2005). Recruitment and retention strategies: A Magnet hospital prevention model. *Medical-Surgical Nursing, 4,* 21–27.

U.S. Citizenship & Immigration Services. (2009). *e-Verify.* Retrieved from http://www.uscis.gov/portal/site/uscis/menuitem.eb1d4c2a3e5b9ac89243c6a7543f6d1a/?vgnextoid=75bce2e261405110VgnVCM1000004718190aRCRD&vgnextchannel=75bce2e261405110VgnVCM1000004718190aRCRD

U.S. Congress. Senate. Committee on Labor and Human Resources. *Conference on the growing contingent work force: Flexibility at the price of fairness?* 103rd Cong., 2d sess., 1994. Available at http://www.archive.org/stream/conferenceongrow00unit/conferenceongrow00unit_djvu.txt

U.S. Department of Health and Human Services. (2009). *Children's Health Insurance Program Reauthorization Act of 2009 overview.* Retrieved from http://www.cms.hhs.gov/home/chip.asp

U.S. Department of Labor. (n.d.-a). *Drug-free workplace policy builder: Section 7: Drug testing.* Retrieved from http://www.dol.gov/elaws/asp/drugfree/drugs/screen92.asp

U. S. Department of Labor. (n.d.-b). *The Fair Labor Standards Act of 1938, as amended.* Retrieved from http://www.dol.gov/whd/fmla/fmlaAmended.htm

U.S. Department of Labor. (n.d.-c). *The Family and Medical Leave Act of 1993, as amended.* Retrieved from http://www.dol.gov/whd/fmla/fmlaAmended.htm

U.S. Department of Labor. (n.d.-d). *FAQs for employees about COBRA continuation health coverage.* Washington, DC: Author. Available online at http://www.dol.gov/ebsa/faqs/faq_consumer_cobra.html

U. S. Department of Health and Human Services. (n.d.-e) *Health information privacy.* Retrieved from http://www.hhs.gov/ocr/privacy/hipaa/understanding/cosumers/index.html

U.S. Department of Labor. (n.d.-f). *Title VII, Civil Rights Act of 1964, as amended.* Retrieved from http://www.dol.gov/oasam/regs/statutes/2000e-16.htm

U.S. Department of Labor. (n.d.-g). *Voluntary safety and health program management guidelines.* Retrieved from http://www.osha.gov/pls/oshaweb/owadisp.show_document?p_table=FACT_SHEETS&p_id=127

U.S. Department of Labor. (n.d.-h) *When can an employee's scheduled hours of work be changed* [e-laws—Fair Labor Standards Act Advisor]. Retrieved from http://www.dol.gov/elaws/faq/esa/flsa/015.htm

U.S. National Archives & Records Administration. (2012). *Our Documents—National Labor Relations Act* (1935). Retrieved from http://www.ourdocuments.gov/doc.php?flash=true&doc=67

U.S. Office of Personnel Management. (n.d). *Patients Bill of Rights.* Retrieved from http://www.opm.gov/insure/health/reference/billrights.asp

U.S. Securities and Exchange Commission. (2012). *The Dodd Frank whistleblower program.* Retrieved from http://www.sec.gov/spotlight/dodd-frank/whistleblower.shtml

Vietnam Era Veterans' Readjustment Assistance Act of 1974 38 U.S.C. § 4212.

CHAPTER 7

THE BUSINESS OF HEALTH CARE

BUDGET

Understanding the budgeting process is a key competency for nurse executives and leaders today. The outcomes of budget management include cost control, market expansion, and a plan for response to current economic trends. The budget is a cooperative effort between the financial department and a responsibility center manager.

A *budget* is a plan for coordinating financial goals of an organization and is a formal quantitative expression of management's plans, intentions, or expectations. A budget provides information that permits executives and managers the ability to develop actions to control results in future reporting periods. It is a quantitative statement, usually expressed in monetary terms, of the plans and expectations of a defined entity (e.g., company, department, unit) over a specified time period.

A budget forces managers to think ahead, compels them to make choices, provides a plan or forecast of what is expected, provides communication within the organization, and provides a basis for evaluation and control. Well-planned budgets determine what needs to be done, when, by whom, and at what cost.

The budgeting process is ongoing, is dynamic, and provides feedback. It is much like the nursing process in that it includes a collection of data from multiple sources, a creation of a plan for activities and services to be delivered, an implementation of the plan, and an evaluation of the outcomes.

Budgets, budget reports, and forecasts are used to demonstrate the fiscal responsibility and financial health of an organization. Generated income is placed in the "trust" of the organization with the assumption that the resources will be used wisely and well for their intended purpose.

Development

Budget information is supplied to managers in advance of the annual budget-planning cycle. The information provides a retrospective history of the financial activities and status of the department, unit, or organization. It also shows the anticipated revenue for the coming year, the revenue sources, and any uncertainties related to revenue streams. Optimistic, moderate, and pessimistic scenarios may be presented as part of the budget development process.

Managers work within a timeline to create preliminary, revised, and final budgets consistent with the practices of the organization. Review and approval procedures are built into the development process all along the line. Therefore, once the final budget is released, there should be no major surprises.

Monitoring

Managers are expected to routinely monitor budget reports. In most cases, reports are generated and reviewed monthly. Managers are asked to justify deviations from the budget predictions and to make adjustments accordingly. In some cases, monthly allocations are divided equally among the months of the year. In other cases, monthly allocations are adjusted on the basis of historical trends. In any case, managers must become familiar with those trends and the trending methodology in use in the organization. Failure to consider trends when making interval adjustments to budgets sometimes results in over- or under-correction of variance and can lead to more difficulties in later months.

Reporting

Managers generally receive monthly, quarterly, annual, and predictive budget reports that help them better manage their units or services. In addition, managers should receive reports detailing the overall financial status of the organization. Reports must be reviewed for accuracy and analyzed for hidden content, that is, to learn the "story" behind the numbers. For example, is a high sick rate on a given unit related to an outbreak of the flu, interpersonal conflict, chronic "short staffing," management practices, or none of the above?

To the extent possible, managers should receive financial reports electronically. Such reports may use a simple spreadsheet approach or may be embedded in a more sophisticated software program. In either case, managers should know how to interpret and manipulate both paper and electronic budget reports as part of their practice.

Justifying

Budget items must be *justified,* that is, the reason for the expenditure must be clearly known and understood, and it must be consistent with the overall objectives and fiscal plan of the organization. Most institutions have a justification process. The sponsor of an anticipated expenditure may be requested to submit a business case to justify the item depending on the scope of that expenditure. The organization then prioritizes requests according to established criteria. In certain circumstances, budget items that initially put the organization or the department into a negative variance are seen as justifiable because the long-term return on investment will ultimately yield financial benefit for the organization.

Variance Analysis

Because budgets are fluid, line items are rarely precisely on target. Thus, variance analysis is an essential part of the budget process. If the variance exceeds a predetermined target, then further investigation is warranted; this occurs whether the variance is positive or negative. Variances may be characterized as volume, efficiency, rate, or non-salary expenditures:

- *Volume variances* in the hospital setting may occur in response to a fluctuation in patient-days.
- *Efficiency variances* in the hospital setting may be expressed in changes from the anticipated hours per patient per day (HPPD).
- *Rate variances* reflect the difference between the budgeted hourly rate and the paid hourly rate.
- *Non-salary expenditure variances* may be caused by changes in patient mix and volume, supply quantities and costs, price paid, or new technology or regulations.

Budget Types: Revenue, Expense, Capital, and Operating

The budget categories that managers deal with on an ongoing basis fall primarily into the following categories: revenue, expense, capital, and operating.

Revenue

Revenue is the total amount of income anticipated during a defined period of time. Income sources include reimbursement for patient care, sales of goods and products, and membership dues in the case of direct-member health maintenance organizations (HMOs).

Revenue generation is rarely under the direct control of managers. A certain percentage of actual or anticipated revenue is allocated to the various cost centers under the manager's direction.

The manager is responsible for operating within the revenue allocation by controlling expenses or creating services that will generate revenue. The extent to which the manager can control fixed expenses is generally limited. Thus, she or he exerts the greatest influence on fiscal stability by controlling variable expenses, including payroll costs (see "Cost Containment," p. 172).

Expense

The *expense* budget is comprised of salary and non-salary items. In general, managers are responsible for managing expenditures within an assigned *cost center* (implies outflow of resources/cash). In some settings, managers may also be responsible for a *profit center* (implies inflow of cash).

Costs are described as fixed and variable:

- *Fixed costs* remain constant for the organization despite fluctuations in activity levels, such as rental fees, contract fees, and insurance premiums.
- *Variable costs* fluctuate in response to some internal or external influence, such as changes in census, patient acuity, staff mix, or product cost.

Capital

The *capital* budget includes equipment and renovation expenses needed to meet long-term goals. Organizations define criteria for items included in the capital budget. In general, these items must have an expected life span (performance) of 1 year or more and exceed a certain dollar value. When budgeting for capital items, costs other than the item itself must be considered, such as installation, delivery charges, and service contracts.

Managers are expected to understand the capital budgeting process for their organization. *Amortization*, an assignment of costs to the capital item for its lifetime, is part of the capital process but often is overlooked by managers during the budgeting process. Knowing the "life expectancy" of equipment, programs, or services is critically important so that a replacement strategy can be built into the capital budgeting process.

While it is not always possible to predict the rate of obsolescence of a given product or to know what replacement technology is on the horizon, it behooves most managers to gain a greater understanding of the capital process than they currently possess. Those managers who do not have a formal background in finance are well advised to develop working relationships with analysts and controllers in the finance department or to take advantage of participation in a formal budget basics course. In this way, managers can gain valuable fiscal management skills.

On a larger scale, capital planning is used to predict and plan for the environmental needs of an organization, that is, the buildings and space the organization requires to conduct its business. The regulatory requirements that surround building plans are such that a relatively long lead time is required. As the delivery of health care and the technology used in its delivery has changed rapidly and significantly in recent years, the traditional planning process has taken on new urgency and faces difficult challenges. In some cases, buildings constructed to house designated clinical services have become outdated even before they are opened because the rate of technology innovation has outstripped the construction schedule.

Operating

The *operating budget,* or annual budget, is based on anticipated revenues and expenses for the organization's fiscal year (12 months, not necessarily in concert with the calendar year). Revenue and expense segments are separated, which allows for easy calculation of "bottom-line" profit or loss. The operating budget is revisited throughout the year to determine if the organization is on target to meet its projected financial goals. Management practices have a significant impact on the operating budget.

Other Terminology

The following budgetary terms are part of the nursing leader's financial lexicon:

- *Assets:* The financial resources an organization receives (i.e., accounts receivable).
- *Break-even point:* The point at which *revenue* (see definition in this list) covers cost. The break-even point can be determined by dividing the *fixed cost* by the *contribution margin*. For example, if the charge for a procedure is $25, and the actual cost of the procedure is $10, the contribution margin is $15. If the fixed cost for the procedure for a given period of time (e.g., 12 months) is $30,000, then it would be necessary to perform 2,000 procedures to break even. Most hospitals have high fixed costs.
- *Capital budget:* Long-range planning tool for organizations; replacement items budgeted under capital generally have a 1- to 5-year life span.
- *Case mix:* The types of patients served by an institution, usually defined by variables such as diagnosis, payment source, personal characteristics, and patterns of treatment.
- *Cash flow:* The rate at which dollars are received and disbursed.

- *Centers for Medicare and Medicaid Services (CMS):* The federal agency responsible for implementing Medicare and Medicaid reimbursement regulations. In its reorganized state, CMS has three distinct areas of responsibility: (1) the Center for Medicare Management, (2) the Center for Beneficiary Choices, and (3) the Center for Medicaid and State Operations.
- *Contribution margin:* Portion of the charge (to a patient) for a procedure or for supplies that is over and above the actual cost and which the cost center contributes to *revenue.* For example, if a procedure costs $10, and the patient is charged $25, the contribution margin is $15. The contribution margin is the profit that is contributed by a cost center *without* the *indirect costs.*
- *Cost–benefit ratio:* Numerical relationship between the value of an activity or procedure in terms of benefits and the value of the activity's cost. The cost–benefit ratio is expressed as a fraction. If the fraction is greater than 1, benefits outweigh costs (i.e., the activity is economically beneficial).
- *Cost center:* Smallest functional unit for which cost control and accountability can be assigned. A nursing unit or floor is usually referred to as a cost center, but there may be other cost centers within a unit (e.g., Orthopedics is a cost center, but often the cast room is considered a separate cost center within Orthopedics).
- *Cost finding:* Process of determining full cost of services or procedures by allocating *indirect costs* and adding them together with *direct costs.*
- *Diagnostic-related groups (DRGs):* Medical classifications under which a Medicare patient's diagnosis will be made. Each DRG has a set payment reimbursement rate. This rate may, in actuality, be higher or lower than the cost of treating a patient in a particular institution.
- *Direct costs:* Costs attributed to a specific source, such as medications and treatments.
- *Endowments:* Resources contributed by a donor but that are held aside to generate additional income for a hospital. For example, a piece of real estate might be donated to a hospital to produce income.
- *Expendable supplies:* Supplies that are consumed as used and therefore are not reusable.
- *Fixed budget:* Style of budgeting based on a fixed annual level of volume, such as number of patient-days or tests performed, to arrive at an annual budget total. Totals are then divided by 12 to arrive at a monthly average. The fixed budget does not make provision for monthly or seasonal variations.
- *Fixed costs:* Costs that do not vary according to volume, such as mortgage or loan payments.
- *Flexible budget:* Budgeting system that takes into account variations in volume. Range of activity is estimated based on a projected range of volume from low to high.
- *Forecasting:* Process by which future activities are translated into resource needs (e.g., persons, supplies, equipment), which are then translated into dollar amounts.
- *Full cost:* Total of all *direct costs* and *indirect costs.*

- *Full-time equivalent (FTE):* Number of hours of work for which a full-time employee is scheduled for a weekly period. For example, 1.0 FTE = 5 8-hour days of staffing, which equals 40 hours of staffing per week. One FTE can be divided in different ways. For example, 2 part-time employees, each working 20 hours per week, would equal 1.0 FTE. If a position requires coverage for more than 5 days or 40 hours a week, the FTE will be greater than 1.0 for that position. If a position requires 7-day coverage for more than 5 days (or 40 hours) a week, the FTE will be greater than 1.0 for that position. If a position requires 7-day coverage, or 56 hours, then that position requires 1.4 FTE coverage (56 divided by 40 = 1.4). If a position requires 7-day coverage or 56 hours, with a 12-hour schedule, the position requires 2.33 FTE coverage (84 divided by 36). This means that more than 1 person is needed to fill the FTE position for a 7-day period.
- *Gross income:* Total income received before expenses are deducted.
- *Health Care Financing Administration (HCFA):* Federal agency responsible for implementing Medicare reimbursement regulations.
- *Hours per patient day (HPPD):* Hours of nursing care provided per patient per day by various levels of nursing personnel. HPPD are determined by dividing total production hours by number of patients.
- *Indirect costs:* Costs that cannot be directly attributed to a specific area, such as housekeeping, and are usually spread among different departments.
- *Inflation factor:* Percentage of rate of inflation. This figure needs to be included in budgeting for the future.
- *Liabilities:* Financial obligations of an organization, such as bills to be paid.
- *Major diagnostic category (MDC):* Major categories under which discreet *DRGs* fall.
- *Master budget:* Total budget for the entire organization, which combines the individual *cost center* budgets.
- *Net income:* Income that remains when expenses have been subtracted from total *revenue.*
- *Net loss:* Loss sustained when expenses exceed total *revenue.*
- *Operating expenses:* Daily costs required to maintain and run a hospital or other healthcare institution.
- *Outliers:* Under the classification of patients by *DRGs,* this term refers to inpatients who are atypical and cannot be classified by DRG.
- *Patient classification system:* Method of classifying patients. Different criteria are used for different systems. In nursing, patients are usually classified according to severity of illness.
- *Planning:* Process by which goals and objectives are set. When planning, it is important to anticipate future problems and to make decisions in advance about how to handle them.
- *Position control plan:* Plan for staffing requirements that determines how many *FTEs* are required to deliver the amount of care identified as being necessary.

- *Preferred provider organization (PPO):* Physician, group of physicians, hospital, or other healthcare facility that has contracted with private insurance companies or individual businesses to provide healthcare services.
- *Production hours:* Total amount of regular time, overtime, and temporary time. This also may be referred to as *actual hours.*
- *Profit margin:* Percentage of difference between expenses and *revenue.*
- *Program budget:* Style of budgeting that involves planning for 5 or 10 years ahead. Attention is paid to external events that might affect an organization. As long-range plans are determined, specific objectives are identified that will lead to the achievement of the plans. The costs required to meet these objectives are then determined. Alternative objectives and their costs also may be identified to provide greater flexibility. Programs are prioritized in order of importance.
- *Restricted resources:* Financial contributions that have restrictions placed on their use by the donor (e.g., resources donated for specific programs, units, services).
- *Revenue:* Items or amounts of income.
- *Semi-fixed costs:* Costs that run at a certain level for a given period of time and then increase. For example, one chef can prepare a certain number of meals at a certain *fixed cost.* After a certain point, another chef needs to be hired to handle the additional volume.
- *Staffing distribution:* Determination of number of personnel allocated per shift (e.g., 45% day shift, 35% evening shift, 20% night shift).
- *Staffing mix:* Ratio of various types of personnel to one another (e.g., a shift on one unit might have 40% RNs, 40% LPNs/LVNs, 20% other personnel).
- *Tax Equity and Fiscal Responsibility Act of 1982* (TEFRA; P.S. 97-248): Federal act that restricted reimbursement to a predetermined rate for Medicare patients. This regulation was superseded in 1984 by the *DRG* method of payment.
- *Turnover rate:* Rate at which employees leave their jobs for reasons other than death or retirement. The rate is calculated by dividing the number of employees leaving by the average number of workers employed in the unit during the year and then multiplying by 100.
- *Unrestricted resources:* Financial contributions that have no restrictions placed on their use by the donor.
- *Variable costs:* Costs that vary with the volume (e.g., payroll costs).
- *Variance:* Difference between planned costs and actual costs.
- *Workload index:* Weighted statistic that reflects acuity level of patients, census, and production hours. This index can serve as a baseline for productivity improvement. One way to determine a workload index is as follows:
    - Acuity Index × Workload Units = Production Hours

- *Zero-based budgeting:* Type of budgeting system that starts at zero each year. This means that every dollar to be spent needs to be justified. Established costs are not automatically continued from one year to the next. This style of budgeting ensures that activities are not continued simply because they were carried out in the past. In zero-based budgeting, objectives are important and are listed according to priority. Zero-based budgeting also indicates what will happen if an objective is eliminated, as well as which objectives could be accomplished for less money (Finkler & Kovner, 2000).

Decision Support Systems

Decision support systems allow managers to make financial decisions and adjustments through computer modeling that uses real-time data. Computer-generated financial forecasting allows organizations to develop alternative scenarios on the basis of the interplay among numerous variables. While computer programs are capable of generating an infinite number of scenarios, it is the wisdom and knowledge of the people in the organization that define the probable scenarios that the organization is likely to face in the near or far term. Astute managers and administrators inform themselves about scenario development, the availability and capability of computerized forecasting systems, and the process used by the organization in forecast planning.

Unlike strategic planning, scenario development is characterized by a focus on *possible* futures. The creation of scenarios allows organizations or departments to compensate for errors common in the planning process—under-prediction and over-prediction. The scenarios create focus on an organization's key concerns in areas of uncertainty.

For example, suppose that the organization's strategic plan predicts 3% to 4% growth over each of the next 10 years and bases its resource acquisition on this assumption. The company faces grave consequences of its financial position if growth falls below 2.6% per year on average. Scenario development will help this company examine the possible consequences of excessive growth or excessive loss, each of which is a possibility and neither of which is accounted for in the strategic plan.

REIMBURSEMENT

Revenue streams for healthcare organizations originate from a variety of sources.

Diagnosis-Related Groups and Prospective Payment Systems

DRGs categorize the care needs of hospitalized patients on the basis of primary and secondary diagnosis, age, and treatments provided. There are over 400 DRGs.

DRGs came into use in 1983 as a way to deter cost shifting within the Medicare system. The DRG reimbursement rate is fixed and is calculated based on the law of averages. The resources used to care for some patients who fall into a particular category will exceed the reimbursement rate; for others, the cost of care will be less than the reimbursement rate.

Medicare's *prospective payment system (PPS)* is the mechanism for transferring funds to hospitals on the basis of the facility's DRG profile. Prospective payment schemes provide a predetermined amount of money to the organization on the basis of the anticipated utilization by a defined group of patients.

While DRGs and PPS were initially a system used by the federal government to constrain Medicare costs, it was merely a matter of time before the process was more widely adopted, first by Medicaid and then by private sector insurers. PPS effectively signaled the end of the "usual and customary" reimbursement system based on *charges* for care or service rather than on the *cost* of those services.

Capitation

Capitation is an inherent part of managed care systems. HMOs, preferred provider organizations (PPOs), and medical service organizations (MSOs) are financed through capitation. Capitation is an integral part of cost-containment efforts under managed care.

In the *capitated model,* the organization is paid a fixed, negotiated rate per member (life covered) per month (PM/PM). The organization receives payment whether or not the member uses the services of the organization in a given time period. Organizations financed under capitation are expected to manage their business in such a way that they provide all needed and agreed-on care to patients covered under the plan.

The business model calls for risk to be spread within the group for the array of services that are agreed to ahead of time. In general, the care provided is "conservative," that is, the services provided are intended to prevent illness, to maintain health, and to care for episodic acute care needs on the basis of known or proven therapies.

The regulations that govern managed care are such that organizations open themselves to considerable risk if they provide care beyond what the plan promises to provide. For example, a request for payment for an experimental treatment that the plan has not yet adopted but that might be of benefit for one member of the plan will be refused. This same treatment may eventually move from experimental to mainstream and be incorporated into the plan's offerings. However, if the plan were to provide the care for the one member who requested it, as noted above, then this same care (i.e., procedure, therapy) would need to be offered to others in the plan with a similar condition. The risk model used by the managed care group is then overridden, placing the organization in financial and regulatory jeopardy.

This is sometimes a difficult concept for the general public to understand, and thus, news headlines tend to place the organization in an unfavorable light. It also is true that some unscrupulous organizations have failed to provide the care and services promised under their capitated contracts.

Health Maintenance Organization

The term *HMO* became part of the healthcare lexicon in 1973 with the passage of the Health Maintenance Organization Act (P.L. 93-222), which established federal standards for HMOs and required companies of a certain size to offer at least one HMO to their employees. The principles underlying HMOs are cost-effectiveness based on productivity; population management with a focus on preventive care; a predetermined and agreed-on array of services, including ambulatory and inpatient care; prepayment in the form of "dues" or "membership;" and assumption of risk by the provider to meet the requirements of the promised care and service.

Prepaid group practice is considered the precursor to HMOs. Prepaid group practices were recommended as long ago as 1932 as the most effective delivery system (Starr, 1984). Insurers, employers, or others contract with the physician group to provide a predetermined range of benefits to a specific population for a fixed and agreed-on price. Providers in this arrangement put themselves at risk in that they were required to provide the full range of agreed-on services, regardless of whether the cost of benefits exceeded the established rate of payment.

Ross-Loos, established in Los Angeles in the 1920s, and Kaiser Permanente, established on the West Coast in the 1930s, are the models for prepaid group practice (Starr, 1984). In their early days, they were considered "outcasts" by the traditional medical establishment. This is no longer the case.

Several HMO models exist, although recent shakeouts in the healthcare industry have seen some insurers exiting the HMO market and some excellent programs becoming insolvent due to financial crises.

- *Independent (or individual) practice association (IPA):* Open-panel system in which individual physicians or the practice association contract to provide care to enrolled members. Physicians retain their right to treat fee-for-service patients. Many IPAs have ceased existence because they were unable to remain financially viable.
- *Staff model:* Majority of physicians are on the staff of and derive their salary from the HMO; physicians on staff are the sole or major source of care for enrollees.
- *Group model:* Single, large multispecialty group that is the sole or major source of care for enrollees; contract is exclusively with one HMO. Because of the similarity in the staff and group models, the label *staff/group model* often is used.
- *Network model:* Two or more group practices contract to care for the majority of patients enrolled in an HMO plan. The physicians are usually able to care for fee-for-service patients as well as HMO patients.

Constraints apply to those who receive care through HMO systems. Unless they are willing to pay out-of-pocket, members receive care from providers who contract with or who are employed by the HMO. The same is true for choice of hospitals. These limits are generally offset by the array of services provided, the relative lower cost of managed care plans, and the reasonable copayments that some patients pay at the point of care.

Market share for HMOs tends to be geographical, with significant penetration in metropolitan areas on the East and West Coasts and in a few markets in the interior, such as Minneapolis/St. Paul. The extent to which managed care will be adopted in other markets is unknown. Through the 1990s, the assumption was that the HMO approach to care would prevail over time (Gabel, 1997). That certainty is no longer apparent in the face of the collapse of respected programs and a growing pessimism within the medical community, most having to do with reimbursement conflicts under various managed care contracts.

Social Health Maintenance Organization

The *social health maintenance organization (SHMO)* is a demonstration model conducted under the sponsorship of Medicare to determine the value and feasibility of combining social, health, and medical services under one umbrella with a single payment. Services provided, in addition to those covered under traditional Medicare or Medicaid, include adult day care, dental, vision, hearing, meals, transportation, hospice care, respite care, homemaker services, and chronic care in a nursing facility without prior hospitalization.

A demonstration project, the Program for All-Inclusive Care for the Elderly, conducted under the auspices of the Health Care Financing Administration (now CMS), replicated the On Lok model in place in San Francisco's Chinatown in several locations throughout the country (Medicare, 2008). The intent was to determine the feasibility of increasing Medicare long-term-care (LTC) benefits. Early findings showed that SHMOs were able to reduce hospitalization rates compared with the rates of the non-SHMO Medicare population, but that total costs were not necessarily reduced. All sites experienced substantial losses during the first 3 years of operation. By year 5, two projects broke even or experienced modest gains; the other two sustained losses.

The SHMO demonstration tests a model of service delivery intended to integrate acute, chronic, and LTC. It has operated since 1985 and been evaluated twice. The Secretary of Health and Human Services submitted the final evaluation report of the SHMO to Congress on February 28, 2003 (CMS, 2009b; Medicare, 2008). The Balanced Budget Refinement Act of 1999 (P.L. 106-113) required the Medicare Payment Advisory Commission (MedPAC or the Commission) to submit recommendations regarding the project to the Congress no later than 6 months after the Secretary submitted the final evaluation report. Two evaluations found no conclusive evidence of positive effects on beneficiary health or functioning (CMS, 2009b; Medicare, 2008). They found that the demonstration did not consistently reduce hospital use or long-term nursing facility use or consistently deliver superior quality care. Any favorable effects on service use and use of preventive care were attributable to general characteristics of tightly organized managed care rather than to the features of the model being tested in the demonstration.

The concern with equity for plans and beneficiaries leads us to conclude that all beneficiaries should be able to receive the same benefit package regardless of where they live and that certain plans should not be advantaged relative to other plans. Equity in payment and coverage policies requires that Medicare treat similar health plans and providers the same unless a payment differential is warranted based on the performance of an organization.

SHMOs are currently paid more than regular Medicare+Choice (M+C) plans and are mandated to provide certain additional services. Because there is no clear evidence that SHMOs improve outcomes or reduce costs and as SHMOs and Medicare+Choice plans enroll similar types of members, converting SHMOs to Medicare+Choice and paying them as M+C plans is appropriate (CMS, 2009b; Medicare, 2008). At its April 2003 public meeting, the Commission agreed to recommend that plans participating in the SHMO demonstration be converted to Medicare+Choice coordinated care plans on December 31, 2003.

Medicare makes risk-adjusted payments to Medicare+Choice plans to improve the accuracy of payments to plans that enroll a cross section of beneficiaries, but refinements may be needed for those plans that concentrate on certain types of enrollees. Thus, the Commission also recommends (MedPAC, 2003) that the Secretary of Health and Human Services study payment adjustments for the frail population in the Medicare+Choice program (CMS, 2009b). There are some indications that the second generation (S/HMO II) model was more effective with frail, medically at-risk enrollees. However, the small number of very frail individuals enrolled in the S/HMO II made it difficult to detect relatively short-term effects on nursing home use or other key outcomes.

Negotiating Capitated Discount Rates

During the budgeting process, healthcare organizations assess various income streams, including a review of *capitated contracts.* In the presence of a guaranteed income for an agreed-on set of services for a given population group, the organization may agree to the payer's request for a discounted rate. Before such an agreement is reached, the organization must determine how much risk it is willing to accept to set the discount rate.

For example, suppose the capitated rate for Group A is set at *X* dollars per member, per month. Group A is considered a moderate risk group, is mixed in age, and has a history of reasonable use of services. Group B, on the other hand, is composed of young, healthy members with very low utilization and no chronicity. The benefits coordinator for Group B wants to negotiate a lower rate, preferably with no increase in co-pays for Group B members. The organization must determine if it can sustain the risk and agree to a steeper discounted rate for Group B. If it does agree in principle, then the copayment issue must still be addressed.

In the current market, "low-rate, high-deductible" products are becoming popular with payers and members alike. Members who opt for these products generally see themselves as being in excellent health and in need of very little healthcare services. They reason, and employers and payers may concur, that the lowest cost plan is their best choice. The decision seems reasonable until such a time as the law of averages takes hold and the healthy individual has a catastrophic accident or experiences an unexpected illness and is faced with a devastatingly high co-pay.

Preferred Provider Organizations

Preferred provider organizations (PPOs) came into being in response to discontent with other models of managed care. The PPO is an integrated system that serves as a broker between the purchaser of care and the provider. In a PPO, clients have the option to use or not use the preferred providers available in the plan. In-plan providers are generally considered more "attractive" to clients because of lower costs and greater benefits. Providers are paid a discounted fee for service and do not participate in financial risk sharing.

Although the PPO affords the client greater choice than a staff model HMO, its ability to control costs is limited by the level of discount that can be negotiated with providers.

Third-Party Payers

Traditional *third-party payers* do not provide any direct care; rather, they pay providers or provider groups to care for defined groups or individuals. The U.S. government is the largest third-party payer; it is the exclusive payer for traditional Medicare and funds Medicaid at varying rates depending on contributions negotiated state by state. A substantial number of Medicare and Medicaid contracts are now negotiated as managed care contracts.

Traditional indemnity insurance offers the greatest freedom and flexibility. Those covered by such a plan can choose to receive care from any primary care or specialist physician or go to the hospital of their choosing at any time. They also can change physicians or hospitals at will. The insurance company pays for the majority of care received in an acute care facility and pays varying amounts for outpatient services depending on the buyer's choice of plan. For example, healthy young people are likely to choose a high deductible plan in which they will pay out-of-pocket for the majority of outpatient care received in a given year. The out-of-pocket costs are offset by the lower insurance premiums. On the other hand, someone who has chronic health problems will choose a lower deductible and pay a higher premium. In some cases, the premiums for people with preexisting health conditions are prohibitively high, or they may not qualify for indemnity insurance at all, even if they are able to pay the premiums. Several insurance companies, for example, Blue Cross/Blue Shield, offer HMO, PPO, and indemnity plans.

Medicare

The Medicare program was created in 1965 through Title XVIII of the Social Security Act (P.L. 89-97) to pay for health services for people ages 65 and older. Although it was initially aimed at the retirement age population (at the time of its passage, age 65 was the mandatory retirement age as well as the age for Social Security eligibility), Medicare was expanded in 1972 to include people of any age with end-stage renal disease (i.e., those receiving dialysis; P.L. 92-603). In 1973, it was expanded to include people of any age who meet Medicare's definition of disability (P.L. 93-66). Ninety percent of Medicare beneficiaries are ages 65 or older (CMS, 2009a). Additional revisions in more recent history include the Medicare Modernization Act of 2003 and the Patient Protection and Affordable Care Act of 2010.

Medicaid

As with Medicare, the Medicaid program was established in 1965 and implemented in 1966. Medicaid is a welfare program that pays for certain mandated health services provided to low-income children and their caretakers. Generally, the caretakers receive, or are eligible to receive, public assistance funds. Until 1996, these funds were administered through Aid to Families with Dependent Children (AFDC; P.L. 74-271). The Personal Responsibility and Work Opportunity Reconciliation Act of 1996 (P.L. 104-93) replaced AFDC with the Temporary Assistance for Needy Families (TANF) program. Over time, amendments to the Medicaid act have been made to include people with developmental disabilities and other low-income groups, including the elderly population, children, and pregnant women (CMS, 2009a).

Medicaid is funded jointly by the federal and state governments. The state's per capita income determines the amount of federal matching funds.

Indemnity Insurance

Indemnity insurance is the traditional method of obtaining health insurance for an array of services that are generally needed only under extraordinary circumstances. Indemnity insurance generally covers a predetermined percentage of acute care services regardless of the absolute charge for those services.

For example, two clients pay the same fixed monthly amount for their insurance on the basis of similarity in their risk factors. One needs a hysterectomy and goes to Hospital A for the procedure. Hospital A charges $2,000 for the care provided. The client's insurance carrier pays 80% of the bill, or $1,600. The client is then responsible for the additional $400. The other client has the same procedure at Hospital B, but the charges are $3,000. Again, the client's insurance carrier pays 80% of the bill, or $2,400, but in this case the client's out-of-pocket expense is $600.

Numerous varieties of indemnity insurance exist. In a "tight" economy that finds employers less willing or able to pay high insurance premiums for employees or in which more people must assume responsibility for their own insurance coverage, low-premium, high-deductible plans are offered as a product line. The impact of such products on the healthcare industry is not yet known.

COST CONTAINMENT

The cost of health care continues to outstrip the rate of inflation by several percentage points each year. The forces that drive costs higher are well known and include the aging of the population and the burden of chronic disease, the cost of technology, the cost of pharmaceuticals, the rising expectations of the public about the capabilities of the healthcare system, and lifestyle choices. In addition, the healthcare industry has lagged in its adoption of efficiencies apparent in other large-scale enterprises. Some industry watchers suggest that healthcare costs could be significantly reduced if the industry applied proven efficiency measures to its practices.

A variety of interventions have been attempted or are in place to staunch the ever-increasing amount spent on health care. The degree to which these measures are succeeding is unknown; "voluntary" measures attempted in the past, such as the professional review organizations, were considered a failure. It is possible that some measures now in place are working even as the cost of care continues to rise. Some analysts suggest that, in the absence of these measures, costs would rise even more rapidly.

Below, briefly outlined, are several approaches to cost containment.

Managed Care

Managed care is an amorphous term, not unlike *quality care*. Still, most would agree that a central concept of managed care is the integration, at some level, of the financing and delivery of care. Patient utilization and provider practices are overseen by an entity that has a fiduciary interest in the interactions between the two. Models of managed care have been described above (e.g., HMOs, SHMOs).

Advocates of managed care expect that it will

- Optimize the use of resources, avoiding overuse or underuse,
- Increase accountability at all levels,
- Accurately predict expenditures,
- Contain or reduce expenditures,
- Shift focus from acute care and crisis intervention to disease prevention and health maintenance,
- Reduce variation in practice, and
- Ensure better outcomes of care.

Full realization of the ideals listed above remains elusive even in the best of managed care systems; progress is slow. To its detractors, the term is regarded with disdain, the concept is considered a failure, and the impact is seen as a "take away."

Value-Based Purchasing

Value-based purchasing—what value is assured to the patient? What value is the patient receiving by purchasing a certain organization's health services? For example, one hospital has one guaranteed price regardless of outcome. A patient has cardiac surgery and develops a sternal wound infection requiring a readmission. There is no additional charge to the patient or the insurance company because there was a guaranteed fixed price.

Accountable Care Organizations (ACOs)

Today, reimbursement generally occurs in silos with separate bills for each type of service. With *accountable care organizations* (ACOs), there is one bill across settings. For example, a woman is diagnosed in primary care with degenerative joint diseases of her hip. She is referred to orthopedics. She has a total hip replacement and then goes to a rehabilitation hospital for intense physical therapy. Following a stay at the rehabilitation hospital, the patient is discharged to home with home physical therapy. With an ACO, there is one bill across all of these settings (bundled building and reimbursement). Generally, the better the quality, the better the reimbursement. A medical home (primary care or a clinic) is an integral part of an ACO.

Cost–Benefit Analysis

Cost–benefit analysis is the process of examining scenarios to determine the relative value of an intervention when measured against predetermined criteria. For example, is it more or less cost-effective to provide home care or to pay for care in a skilled nursing facility? Is it more or less cost-effective to care for indigent patients in the emergency department than to establish a community clinic? Though the answers to these dilemmas may seem intuitive, they are not; nor is the process of analysis, because human lives are at stake and the emotions of the decision-makers, not to mention of the target populations, come into play.

While traditional cost–benefit analysis techniques have been used in health care for many years, more sophisticated systems are now being introduced. One such approach is the Archimedes simulation model (Kaiser Permanente, 2009), which represents physiological, clinical, and administrative events as they occur in reality. Archimedes includes all aspects of care—faculties, personnel, care processes, protocols, logistics and costs, multiple disease conditions, and needed interventions over time.

Biomathematical modeling allows analysts to address complex problems rapidly and inexpensively, in contrast to other methods such as clinical trials, observational studies, or the judgment of experts. The extent to which biomathematical modeling achieves its promise is yet to be determined.

Productivity

Productivity is an industrial term that describes the relationship between *outputs* (products delivered) and *inputs* (the resources used to produce the outputs). Whether or not the traditional concept of productivity can be applied to complex systems such as health care remains a subject for debate.

The Agency for Healthcare Research and Quality (AHRQ), formerly known as the Agency for Healthcare Policy and Research (AHCPR), commissioned Patient Outcome Research Teams (PORTs) to answer critical questions about the effectiveness and cost-effectiveness of available treatments for common clinical conditions (AHRQ, 2009a). Beginning in 1989, the AHCPR funded the PORTs, 14 projects that were succeeded, starting in 1993, by a "second generation" of projects known as PORT–IIs. Together, the PORTs and PORT–IIs represent a total investment of more than $100 million to answer critical questions about the effectiveness and cost-effectiveness of available treatments for common clinical conditions.

The PORTs were designed to take advantage of readily available data and to focus on common clinical conditions that are costly to the Medicare and Medicaid programs and for which there is regional variability in outcomes and use of resources. The PORTs were made up of a multidisciplinary team of researchers ranging from health economists and clinicians to quality-of-life experts and epidemiologists. PORT investigators were instructed to answer the following questions: What works and at what cost? For which patients or subgroups of patients? When? Why is there variation in the use of treatments? What can be done to reduce inappropriate variation? From whose perspective (i.e., The patient is the ultimate judge of effectiveness? Is there a potential for development and use of patient-reported outcome measures?)

Specific to nursing, two models of productivity are briefly described here: (1) the industrial model and (2) the systems framework.

The *industrial model* measures the ratio of work output to work input (i.e., efficiency). Nursing HPPD or costs per unit of service are examples of the industrial model on the basis of principles of the school of scientific management that came into its own in the 1920s (see Chapter 2).

The *systems framework* embraces both efficiency and effectiveness. In this model, *effectiveness* includes quality and appropriateness; *efficiency* includes nursing output with minimal waste. This model takes into consideration the special characteristics of nursing, such as caring.

- *Nursing HPPD* = Divide total paid hours for nursing personnel for a specific time period by the total number of patient days in the same time period.
- *Salary costs per patient per day* = Divide total payroll expenses for nursing personnel for a specific time by the total number of patient days in the same time frame (more sensitive measure than HPPD in that it accounts for staff mix).
- *Utilization rate* = Divide required hours of care by nursing hours paid (more sensitive in that hours of care required are based on a patient classification system; results show differences, if any, between the required and actual staffing ratios).

Patient/Client Classification

Classification systems assign patients to defined categories by care intensity, care level, assumed or average utilization of resources, or other variables.

Healthcare systems may devise their own patient classification systems; however, the tools they use must be valid and reliable. Alternatively, several commercial classification systems are readily available for purchase. The purchase of an acuity system package is accompanied by support service from the product's creator or vendor. All commonly available acuity systems are automated.

DRGs, as discussed earlier in this chapter, are actually a classification system related to reimbursement based on intensity of need. DRG/PPS was initially applied to care provided for Medicare patients in acute care hospitals and was based on the projected case mix for the institution, adjusted for age. Other payers, including Medicaid and then the private sector, adopted Medicare's approach. PPS has expanded over time and is now applied in other healthcare settings such as skilled nursing facilities.

PPS was instituted to deter cost-shifting. The practice of *cost-shifting* allowed hospitals to recover some uncompensated billings by transferring these costs to Medicare and other payers. With cost-shifting no longer an option, hospitals needed to cut costs to continue to operate. The intervening years have seen a large number of hospital closures and consolidation throughout the industry.

An entire sub-industry has developed in response to DRGs. Coders, case management enterprises, nurses who specialize in discharge planning and patient placement, publishing companies that produce DRG manuals, and designated government departments now exist to ensure compliance with PPS regulations.

Savings related to the advent of DRGs are generally attributed to two factors: (1) decreased lengths of stay in acute care facilities and (2) avoidance of admissions when care can be provided safely in another setting. Establishing a link between DRG classifications and nursing acuity classification is a challenging but worthwhile endeavor.

Staff Mix

The pattern of assigning defined categories of staff to care for a specific group of patients is known as *staff mix*. The staff mix may be more or less heavily weighted toward the use of registered nurses (RNs), depending on the philosophy of the institution. RNs, licensed practical/vocational nurses, and unlicensed assistive personnel (e.g., nurse aides) make up the bulk of a hospital's staff mix for direct care. Other disciplines may assist in the provision of direct or indirect care.

Staffing ratios relative to the use of RNs may be prescribed by legislation, particularly for specialty areas such as intensive care units. RN ratio legislation for other care settings now exists in some states, a trend that is likely to prevail in the coming years. For example, former California Governor Gray Davis signed into law a bill mandating minimum nurse-to-patient staffing ratios (Mentz, 2008). Despite legislative intent and institutional commitment, the extent to which staff ratios can be met depends on the availability of RNs. The current nursing shortage is predicted to worsen, at least in the near term.

Critics of staffing ratios maintain that this approach alone is an insufficient guarantee of safe care. Rather, the patient's overall condition, intensity of needs, and requisite competence of the staff must be considered when determining the optimum staff mix for a particular service (Dilcher, 1999).

Reduction in Staff and Services

Costs can be contained through *reduction in force (RIF)* strategies and the cutback or elimination of services not seen as critical to the organization's goals, including that of maintaining fiscal viability. *Outsourcing* is another approach to cost reduction. Competitive bids for certain services can be obtained and vendors selected for such services as housekeeping, food, linen, and the like. Payroll, transcription, and other business services can be contracted. *Temporary agencies* can be used to supplement core staffing, particularly to meet seasonal needs. The relatively high per hour cost of temporary employees may be offset by avoidance of benefit costs. However, cost savings achieved by RIFs may not be sustained, and hidden costs may outstrip anticipated savings.

Ethical, legal, and contractual issues must be considered when RIFs occur. Can the organization's ethical commitment to safe patient care be maintained in the face of downsizing? Does the organization place itself in harm's way by inviting sanctions from regulatory agencies if preventable violations occur? Do contracts include "no-layoff" clauses for members of organized labor who may staff the organization?

Material Management

Economists, efficiency experts, administrators, and frontline staff generally agree that resources can be better managed through the development and application of better business, information, and care systems. In the abstract, there are no arguments about the need to decrease waste in the delivery of health care. Controlling the cost of supplies and equipment is a never-ending challenge for managers and staff. The process of competitive bidding allows organizations to obtain significant discounts on quality products from various vendors or distributors. While this practice is beneficial to the organization overall, it also tends to isolate staff from the actual cost of materials and supplies in that the cost to the organization is generally closely held information (for good reason).

Inventory control systems help match supply and demand, may decrease utilization, and may decrease loss due to theft. "Pricing" frequently used items may help staff "comparison shop" for the most cost-effective products and supplies even within their own department or institution. Compared with other industries, healthcare inventory control systems are still on the upward curve of the improvement process. In the past, supply costs were "passed through" and reimbursed through the third-party system. Patients as well as staff remained immune to the cost of supplies which, when itemized, also include the cost of processing.

As with salary and non-payroll personnel costs, managers receive monthly reports detailing materials costs for their units or departments.

MARKETING

Purpose, Market Share, Penetration, and Mix

The purpose of marketing is to identify customer needs and meet them in a way that returns value to the organization. The business approach to marketing was once anathema to health care. However, healthcare organizations must market their products and services through usual marketing channels such as advertising and direct-to-consumer approaches to create a new and repetitive customer base (Chang, Price, & Pfoutz, 2001).

The *four P* approach to marketing includes *p*roduct, *p*ricing, *p*lace, and *p*romotion to today's marketing orientation. Effective marketing orientation also is called *customer orientation,* which focuses energy on identifying the wants and needs of consumers and on delivering services that create satisfaction (Alward & Camunas, 1991).

Through market analysis, healthcare establishments can determine the existence of potential customers and their needs, the products and services that appeal to target groups, the status of and techniques used by competitors (*benchmarking*), and what price the market will bear (although there are constraints in this last element for most players in the healthcare market). An organization's *market share* is the percentage of the total available market for product or service that is captured by producer or organization.

Market penetration refers to how well the organization has exposed its services to potential users or buyers. Are the potential buyers aware of the organization, of its products and services, of the price of the products and services—and are the products and services appealing to those potential customers? Market share is that portion of the market that is supplied by the organization (e.g., how many "lives" a particular provider covers).

A *market mix* is an organization's individualized blend of marketing tools and tactics implemented to achieve its goals. The term also can be applied to the variety and scope of the products or services the organization has to offer to its potential market.

Advertising and the Media

Brand recognition happens through advertising. *Brand loyalty* is sustained through advertising. Traditional advertising modalities such as newspapers, television (including "infomercials"), and radio are expensive. Thus, healthcare organizations exercise discretion when making decisions to purchase advertising time and space. Most organizations take advantage of "free" publicity (e.g., public interest stories that shed a positive light on the organization). Organizations also plan for and evaluate the effectiveness of their advertising campaigns through techniques such as focus groups, surveys, and interviews.

The majority of hospitals and healthcare systems have a presence on the Internet. They, along with other healthcare entities that use the Internet to share information, subscribe to the IHealth Code of Ethics. IHealth's vision statement is

> The goal of the IHealth Code of Ethics is to ensure that people worldwide can confidently and with full understanding of known risks realize the potential of the Internet in managing their own health and the health of those in their care. (Rippen & Risk, 2000)

Values expressed in the code include candor and honesty; quality of information, products, and services; respect for individuals' right to give informed consent; and respect for privacy and protection of confidential information.

Surveys

An abundance of market research is available to organizations. Most organizations rely on standard market information in addition to their own surveys, usually aimed at brand recognition or identification. Well-structured, professionally conducted focus groups often provide organizations with useful information that allows them to better target subsequent survey activities.

Image Building

Organizations at Large

Most organizations have an image they wish to project, and it must be believable, sustainable, honest, and appealing. The image should foster loyalty among those who are already part of the organization or who obtain services from the organization. It should increase the organization's share of target markets. Once the decision is made to foster a particular image, executive-level efforts should be directed toward ensuring that everyone is "on board" with regard to the organization's public persona.

Nursing

Nurses enjoy a highly favorable image among the public at large. However, the public's image of the nurse is still, in many cases, that of a subservient woman who does the bidding of others. The current nursing shortage actually allows nurses to demonstrate the variety, complexity, and significance of their many roles. Interestingly enough, it is somewhat difficult to describe the deep value of nursing to a general audience, but the challenge is there, and the time to meet it as a profession is now.

Corporations and Foundations

Johnson & Johnson, through its corporate advertising program and through its philanthropic arm, and the Robert Wood Johnson Foundation are promoting the image and value of nursing to a variety of audiences with the intent of helping to alleviate the serious nursing shortage. They put up a website, Discover Nursing (www.discovernursing.com), to help promote the profession.

Public Relations

Organizations employ public relations professionals who interface with the press, various community constituencies, law enforcement, regulatory bodies, employees, and patients and families. Their role is to ensure consistency in the messages sent to those outside of the organization, to prevent jeopardy to the organization, and to serve as the public voice of the organization in a manner that is seen as enthusiastic, positive, and respectful.

Public relations personnel are sometimes called on to do "damage control" and must be prepared to absorb or deflect negative comments while maintaining personal dignity and respect for others, even detractors.

REFERENCES

Agency for Healthcare Research and Quality. (2009a). *HCUP-US overview.* Retrieved from http://www.hcup-us.ahrq.gov/overview.jsp

Agency for Healthcare Research and Quality. (2009b). *Quality and patient safety.* Retrieved from http://www.ahrg.gov/qual

Alward, R., & Camunas, C. (1991). *The nurses' guide to marketing.* Albany, NY: Delmar.

Barton, P. (2003). *Understanding the U.S. health services system* (2nd ed.). Chicago: Health Administration Press.

Centers for Medicare and Medicaid Services. (2002). *Evaluation results for the social/health maintenance organization II demonstration.* Retrieved from http://www.cms.gov/Medicare/Demonstration-Projects/DemoProjectsEvalRpts/downloads/SHMO_Report.pdf

Centers for Medicare and Medicaid Services. (2009a). *Overview Medicaid program.* Retrieved from http://www.cms.hhs.gov/home/medicaid.asp

Centers for Medicare and Medicaid Services. (2009b). *Overview program of All-Inclusive Care for the Elderly (PACE).* Retrieved from http://www.cms.hhs.gov/PACE

Chang, C. F., Price, S. A., & Pfoutz, S. K. (2001). *Economics and nursing: Critical professional issues.* Philadelphia: F.A. Davis.

Cowan, C. A., & Hartman, M. B. (2005). Financing health care: Businesses, household, and governments, 1879–2003. *Health Care Financing Review, 1*(2), 1–26.

Dilcher, A. (1999). *Legislating nurse-to-patient ratios: California legislation falls short.* Retrieved from http://www.law.uh.edu/healthlaw/perspectives/MedicalProfessionals/991019Nurse.html

Finkler, S. A., & Kovner, C. T. (2000). *Financial management for nurse managers and executives* (2nd ed.). Philadelphia: W. B. Saunders.

Gabel, J. (1997). Ten ways HMOs have changed during the 1990s. *Health Affairs, 16*(3), 134–145.

Health Insurance Portability and Accountability and Accessibility Act of 1996, P.L. 104-191, 110 Stat. 1936.

Huber, D. (2006). *Leadership and nursing care management* (3rd ed.). Philadelphia: Saunders/Elsevier.

Kaiser Permanente. (2009). *What is the Archimedes Model?* Retrieved from http://archimedesmodel.com/archimedesmodel.html

Kaplan, T. (1998). *The Tylenol crisis: How effective public relations saved Johnson & Johnson.* Retrieved from http://www.aerobiologicalengineering.com/wxk116/TylenolMurders/crisis.html

Keehan , S., Sisko, A., Truffer, C., Smith, S., Cowan, C., Poisal, J., et al. (2008, February 21). Health spending projections through 2017. *Health Affairs Web Exclusive,* W146.

Medicare. (2008). *Program of All-Inclusive Care for the Elderly (PACE).* Retrieved from http://www.medicare.gov/Nursing/Alternatives/Pace.asp

MedPAC. (2003, August). *Social health maintenance organization (S/HMO): Recommendations for the future of the demonstration* [Report to the Congress]. Retrieved from http://www.medpac.gov/publications/congressional_reports/Aug03_SHMO%20Report.pdf

Mentz, P. (2008). *The original bill that put staffing ratios in place.* Retrieved from http://www.nursetraveler.org/CA-np-ratio.html

Price Waterhouse Cooper. (2002, April). *The factors fueling rising healthcare costs* [Study prepared for the American Association of Health Plans]. Washington, DC: Author.

Rippen, H. & Risk, A. (2000, Apr–Jun). e-Health: Code of Ethics. *Journal of Medical Internet Research, 2*(2). Retreieved from http://www.ncbi.nlm.nih.gov/pmc/articles/PMC1761853/

Starr, P. (1984). *The social transformation of American medicine: The rise of a sovereign profession and making of a vast industry.* New York: Basic Books.

Title 1 Quality Affordable Health Care Bill Title 1 Amendments. Retrieved from http://dpc.senate.gov/healthreformbill/healthbill52.pdf

Yoder-Wise, P. S., & Kowalski, K. E. (2006). *Beyond leading and managing: Nursing administration for the future.* St. Louis, MO: Mosby.

APPENDIX A

REVIEW QUESTIONS

1. In assessing the philosophy for nursing services for possible revision, the nurse executive is most heavily influenced by the organization's:

    a. mission statement.

    b. consumer surveys.

    c. financial resources.

    d. policy statements.

2. In planning for change, the successful change agent under Kurt Lewin's theory makes a commitment to:

    a. help followers arrive at total consensus regarding the change.

    b. encourage subgroup opposition to change so many viewpoints can be heard.

    c. utilize change by drift if resistance to change is too strong.

    d. be available to support those affected by change until refreezing occurs.

3. Strategic planning:

    a. focuses on the long-range goals for the organization.

    b. requires a broad range of management expertise.

    c. is synonymous with tactical planning.

    d. is generally a middle-management function.

4. In planning for managed care, which of the following goals would be most appropriate for the nurse manager?

    a. Clinical outcomes should occur within a prescribed time frame.

    b. Case managers should not function as providers of patient care.

    c. Managed care practice should be unit-based and unit-specific.

    d. Outcome management should be carried out for each patient.

5. Critical pathways outline a patient's expected progress from admission to discharge and are part of

    a. functional nursing.

    b. primary care nursing.

    c. case management.

    d. team nursing.

6. When using a patient classification system, the nurse executive should understand that such systems:

    a. are used to solve unit staffing shortages.
    b. use nonvariable nursing care hours.
    c. are designed to eliminate human error.
    d. are periodically reevaluated.

7. When evaluating the nursing service philosophy, the most important thing to ascertain is that the philosophy:

    a. is congruent with the mission of the organization.
    b. can be implemented in a cost-effective manner.
    c. flows from organizational goals.
    d. is brief and simply worded.

8. In the patient care delivery model of ______________ ______________ ____________, the goal is to work collaboratively with the patient in order to effect a positive outcome.

    a. family-based care
    b. primary nursing care
    c. relationship-based care
    d. differentiated patient care

9. Healthcare professionals have formed a state coalition to propose legislation to change the state's nurse practice act. Controversies have surfaced regarding entry into nursing practice, the role of the licensed practical nurse, and the definition of professional nursing. To communicate information about the proposed changes, it would be most effective for the coalition to:

    a. form a network of all categories of nurses in the state.
    b. mail minutes from coalition group meetings to all constituencies.
    c. work with groups that have lobbied in the past for changes in the nurse practice act.
    d. request that coalition members put the proposed changes on the meeting agendas of other groups to which they belong.

10. The nurse executive attends all high-level meetings. However, he or she seems to have limited access to the organization's true power base and believes there is inequitable distribution of power among executives of the same rank. To change this situation, the nurse executive's most appropriate first step would be to:

    a. propose a plan for organizational restructuring.
    b. form a coalition within the organization to extend her or his network of power.
    c. improve her or his power base by creating a useful level of tension and competition.
    d. become sensitive to informal lines of communication in order to gain entry into informal power groups.

11. The relationship between the operating room nurses and the surgical nurses at a large hospital has become competitive and uncooperative. The focus of the conflict is patient arrival times at the operating room. The nurse executive appoints a performance improvement team to resolve the conflict. Which of the following statements, if made by a team member, would best indicate that progress has been made toward conflict resolution?

    a. "I think it's pretty clear that some people are more responsible than others for this problem."
    b. "I think we should keep exact records of the time factors for 1 month. Then we will know where the discrepancy lies."
    c. "I hadn't realized how much time is involved in preparing patients for surgery."
    d. "It's always good to be able to vent your feelings. It helps when you can tell people what you think."

12. In evaluating the nursing administration's philosophy statement, the nurse executive's most important step would be to:

    a. assess whether the statement provides for flexibility.
    b. assess whether there is consistency between the statement and actual practice.
    c. create a task force of registered nurses to review the statement.
    d. solicit input from peers about the statement's relevance.

13. The nurse executive at a hospital maintains contracts with affiliated educational institutions whose nursing students want to acquire clinical experience. The nurse executive should ensure that each contract includes a:

    a. copy of the nursing program curriculum.
    b. provision that all nursing faculty members be licensed.
    c. provision that each student carry individual malpractice insurance.
    d. provision that the hospital's nursing department retains responsibility for nursing care provided by the students.

14. Which of the following use of limited resources would most likely result in increased reimbursement revenues? Increasing the:

    a. number of clinical nurse specialists.
    b. educational paid days for licensed staff.
    c. educational programs on documentation.
    d. mix and number of clinical staff.

15. Accountable care organizations support integrated care delivery across a continuum of patient care services and support:

    a. individual billing and reimbursement practices.
    b. bundled billing and reimbursement practices.
    c. one-part payer systems.
    d. national health service reimbursement.

16. In attempting to reduce costs, the nurse executive should remember that the largest share of financial resources will be found in

    a. short-term capital acquisitions.
    b. operating costs.
    c. supplies and equipment.
    d. personnel costs.

17. All department heads are required to re-justify their fiscal needs annually during the budget cycle. Budget allocations are made accordingly. This is a description of which of the following types of budgeting?

    a. Incremental budgeting
    b. Perpetual budgeting
    c. Zero-based budgeting
    d. Managed care budgeting

18. The nurse executive who is implementing a hospital's cost-containment program should realize that the most important step is to:

    a. develop an inservice curriculum that focuses on cost containment.
    b. develop methods for determining nursing care costs for each patient category.
    c. negotiate redistribution of non-nursing tasks to other departments.
    d. ask nurses to become a part of the decision-making process in the areas of patient care, unit management, and hospital governance.

19. Costs per unit of service will increase as

    a. volume decreases below the break-even point.
    b. volume increases.
    c. acuity increases.
    d. management turnover occurs.

20. When nurse executives examine job classifications as they plan salary adjustments, they must remember that there are equal-pay tests that must be met to justify such determinations. Therefore, they would examine jobs for which of the following?

    a. Equal danger on the job, equal intelligence for hire, equal responsibility, and identical working conditions
    b. Equal skill, equal effort, equal responsibility, and similar working conditions
    c. Equal job requirements, same working conditions, equal job duties, and equal responsibilities
    d. Equal effort, equal working conditions, identical job duties, and equal job requirements

21. The most common challenge to Title VII of the Civil Rights Act of 1964 is a potential employee's:

    a. arrest record.
    b. nationality.
    c. pregnancy plans.
    d. religious beliefs and practices.

22. Employee rights include the right to a safe and healthy work environment and the right to participate in activities to ensure their protection from job hazards under the:

    a. Fair Labor Standards Act
    b. Equal Employment Opportunities Commission
    c. Occupational Safety and Health Act
    d. American with Disabilities Act

23. Of the following activities, which would be the most important for the nurse executive to personally carry out?

    a. Serve on the policy and procedure committee
    b. Interpret the job description for a newly hired registered nurse
    c. Facilitate the dissemination of research in nursing and management systems
    d. Review the orientation schedule for newly graduated registered nurses

24. A staff nurse at a unionized agency reports that overtime pay for an after-duty class requiring mandatory attendance was coded as straight pay instead of time-and-one-half as called for in the union contract. Unit managers certify the type and amount of overtime pay. Appropriate action by the nurse executive would be to:

    a. follow up with the nurse's manager to make certain she or he is familiar with the contractual overtime requirements.
    b. accompany the nurse to the payroll office and tell them to make the adjustment.
    c. request that the nurse file a grievance so that payroll adjustment can occur.
    d. turn the matter over to the personnel department for corrective action.

25. The union contract in the facility where you are a manager requires that discipline be progressive in all areas except for substance abuse and theft. When an employee commits a first offense of not coming to work as scheduled and neglecting to notify anyone regarding the absence, you would:

    a. give the employee a written reprimand.
    b. counsel the employee verbally (oral warning).
    c. suspend the employee with pay.
    d. suspend the employee without pay.

26. A labor union is attempting to organize the employees of an institution. It would be considered an unfair labor practice if management:

    a. removed outside organizers from the institution's premises.
    b. refused to allow employees to attend a meeting held by labor organizers during work hours.
    c. supplied the union with information requested about specific employees of the institution.
    d. told employees that the nurse executive would rather deal directly with them than with the union when differences arise.

27. Despite the patient's family's requests to the contrary, Dr. Huang writes a "Do not resuscitate" order on Mrs. Bosko's chart following a conversation with the patient in which Dr. Huang affirmed the patient's wishes to forgo life-prolonging intervention in the presence of end-stage renal disease. The predominant ethical principle evident in this case is

    a. beneficence.
    b. autonomy.
    c. justice.
    d. veracity.

28. The predominant ethical belief underlying the requirements of the Health Insurance Portability and Accountability Act (HIPAA) is that of

    a. truth-telling (veracity).
    b. confidentiality.
    c. utility.
    d. autonomy.

29. In terms of professional ethics, the nurse executive is responsible for ensuring that

    a. ethics education programs are provided for the nursing staff on an ongoing basis.
    b. a nursing ethics committee is convened and meets regularly.
    c. each nurse in provided with a copy of the *Code for Nurses with Interpretive Statements* published by the American Nurses Association.
    d. nursing's perspective is represented in the organization's formal mechanisms for addressing ethical dilemmas.

30. Under Title VII of the Civil Rights Act, the employer
    a. is not responsible for discrimination on the part of individual supervisors.
    b. is responsible for discrimination on the part of individual supervisors.
    c. can terminate a supervisor for practices determined to be discriminatory.
    d. can sue the individual supervisor to recover monetary loss suffered because of discrimination settlements against the organization because of a supervisor's behavior.

31. A physician who performs a procedure upon a patient without proper consent has committed
    a. assault.
    b. invasion of privacy.
    c. battery.
    d. false imprisonment.

32. This federal piece of legislation prevents discrimination during a job interview where interviewers can and cannot ask certain questions. The name of this piece of legislation is
    a. Hill-Burton Act
    b. Fair Labor Standards Act
    c. Title VII of the Civil Rights Act of 1964
    d. Hospital Survey and Construction Act

33. The duty to select members of a hospital's medical staff is legally vested in
    a. the governing board.
    b. the chief of staff.
    c. the administration.
    d. the executive committee.

34. The physician–patient relationship may be established by
    a. an expressed or implied contract.
    b. a written contract, witnessed and notarized.
    c. consultation or abandonment.
    d. punitive damages.

35. A physician who promises to use a certain procedure in performing an operation and uses a different procedure instead may be liable for

    a. negligence.
    b. invasion of privacy.
    c. breach of contract.
    d. libel.

36. Carter, a physician specializing in internal medicine, treated Jones for a broken arm. Should Jones later bring a suit for malpractice, Carter will be held liable to the standard of care required for

    a. his specialty.
    b. the specialty in which he was treating Jones.
    c. a general practitioner.
    d. ordinary medical care.

37. The authority to license healthcare practitioners is found in the regulating power of the

    a. individual hospital.
    b. appropriate training program.
    c. state.
    d. licensing board.

38. Nurse executives have a responsibility to know and understand legislation affecting nursing practice in order to:

    a. prevent administrative personnel malpractice actions.
    b. respond quickly and appropriately to necessary changes in nursing services.
    c. protect the organization from lawsuits.
    d. ensure that procedures in nursing practice are carried out correctly.

39. The legal boundaries of nursing practice are defined in each state by the:

    a. American Nurses Association's *Code for Nurses.*
    b. American Nurses Association's standards of practice.
    c. state board of registered nurses.
    d. state nurse practice act.

40. Currently, your agency has policies and procedures in place that meet state requirements for personnel handling toxic substances. The federal government recently adopted a new requirement regarding these substances. It will not be necessary to make changes in nursing service policy and procedure at your agency because the

    a. nurses in your agency have received recent instructions and education in handling these agents.
    b. environmental control officer in your agency has informed you that it is not necessary.
    c. state in which your agency is located has another, more restrictive policy than the new federal policy.
    d. board of directors and chief administrative officer of your agency told you to ignore the policy.

41. With regard to nonprofit institutions, labor–management relations laws, such as the Federal Labor Relations Act,

    a. have no bearing on the relationship between labor and management.
    b. apply in the nonprofit sector in the same way they apply in the for-profit sector.
    c. are modified for nonprofits compared with their application in for-profit organizations.
    d. are irrelevant in a unionized organization.

42. The Americans with Disabilities Act

    a. applies exclusively to those with physical disabilities.
    b. applies only to companies with 25 or more employees.
    c. applies to those whose mental or physical impairment limits one or more major life activities.
    d. sets limits on "reasonable accommodation."

43. Appreciative inquiry is a contemporary approach to foster change by focusing on an organization's best attributes and practices. Appreciative inquiry as a soft business strategy can result in the:

    a. creation of new organizational visions.
    b. disruption of daily operations.
    c. depletion of fiscal resources.
    d. development of new services based on industry trends.

44. Leveraging diversity requires a nurse executive to

    a. create an affirmative action policy to support hiring practices.
    b. be culturally competent in the cultures of all employees.
    c. maximize all talents and intellectual capital within an organization.
    d. develop a restricted policy to only promote from within.

45. Negotiation skills for the nurse executive include:

    a. active listening and attention to nonverbal cues.
    b. knowledge of consensus group problem solving techniques.
    c. ability to negotiate a resolution in only one meeting.
    d. discussing the "bottom line" at the onset of the negotiations.

46. Crisis management objectives include reducing tension during the incident, controlling the flow and accuracy of information, and

    a. increasing operational capacity.
    b. managing resources effectively.
    c. operating in a normal fashion.
    d. focusing on the short-term effects of the crisis.

47. The use of business plans in health care is on the rise. The purpose of a business plan is to:

    a. follow the trend of industry and retail sales.
    b. answer important questions before money is spent.
    c. defend a project or program after the implementation.
    d. become the final marketing guide for the project or program.

48. Behaviors that support organizational transparency include employee access to information, participation in organization initiatives, and:

    a. access to proprietary secrets.
    b. changing to a matrix organizational structure.
    c. collective bargaining.
    d. participation in decision-making.

49. The Fair Labor Standards Act ensures that employees are paid a fair minimum wage, that records of work hours are kept, and that compensation for time worked be paid in

    a. organization IOUs.
    b. cash or check.
    c. stocks or bonds.
    d. Treasury notes.

50. An objective performance appraisal using a graphic rating scale lists behaviors and classifies behaviors on a Likert scale response. A graphic rating scale for a performance appraisal may be incomplete if the scale lacks

    a. explanatory notes for the rating.
    b. a peer review.
    c. a patient satisfaction survey.
    d. personal anecdotal notes.

APPENDIX B

ANSWERS TO THE REVIEW QUESTIONS

1. **Correct Answer: A.** The organization's philosophy must always be consistent with the mission of the enterprise. In this way, there is clarity of intent about what the organization stands for and what it intends to accomplish.

2. **Correct Answer: D.** Without support until the desired change has replaced the status quo, the likelihood of "backsliding" is high. The successful change agent recognizes the need to help her or his clients remain with the process until the desired change has replaced the prior way of doing things.

3. **Correct Answer: A.** Strategic planning, in contrast to tactical planning, is future-directed and concerned primarily with putting in place the resources to achieve long-term goals.

4. **Correct Answer: A.** Evidence-based care trajectories with defined outcomes should be used to effectively and efficiently manage the care of most patients with a given diagnosis or condition.

5. **Correct Answer: C.** Critical pathways are inherent in the case management approach to care and guide care across the continuum.

6. **Correct Answer: D.** The dynamic nature of health care, changing patient characteristics, the introduction of new technology, and so forth, require that nursing departments periodically review the current patient classification process.

7. **Correct Answer: A.** Congruency among the organization's mission, vision, philosophy, goals, and objectives is essential to the success of the entity.

8. **Correct Answer: C.** Relationships are established with the patient. The goal is to work collaboratively with the patient to effect a positive outcome.

9. **Correct Answer: A.** This step will reach the widest audience and generate the greatest response. The network concept also allows for connectivity and relatively quick dissemination of information.

10. **Correct Answer: D.** Greater awareness of the informal structure and the power within it will help the nurse executive strategize in such a way that she or he can improve her or his base of support within the organization.

11. **Correct Answer: C.** This statement shows an awareness of the importance of data gathering and analysis. This person is beginning to understand the performance improvement process.

12. **Correct Answer: B.** The reputation and integrity of the organization is judged by the consistency between its stated philosophy and its actual practices.

13. **Correct Answer: D.** Ensuring that the hospital retains responsibility for patient care ensures accountability and is consistent with the hospital's regulatory requirements.

14. **Correct Answer: C.** Adequate documentation of patient acuity and complexity may translate to better reimbursement for the organization. Reimbursement processes such as prospective payment (diagnostic-related groups) are adjusted for acuity. Coders rely on the accuracy and adequacy of clinicians' documentation to code correctly.

15. **Correct Answer: B.** Accountable care organizations support bundling billing and reimbursement practices. There is one bill across settings.

16. **Correct Answer: D.** The largest line item in a healthcare organization's budget is personnel. This is also the most malleable item and lends itself to up and down adjustments in response to or in anticipation of changes in the financial status of an organization.

17. **Correct Answer: C.** The zero-based budgeting approach asks managers and department heads to begin each budget year with a clean slate and to justify expenditures accordingly.

18. **Correct Answer: B.** Knowing the specific cost of care for various patient categories gives the nurse executive, along with others within the department, the needed knowledge upon which to base a cost-containment plan.

19. **Correct Answer: A.** This model is based on the premise that a certain volume is needed to maintain cost balance. When the volume decreases below the break-even point, costs go up. For example, staffing for a 50-bed unit is calculated for an occupancy rate of 85%, with a break-even point of 80%. Downward adjustments in staff numbers occur only when the occupancy rate dips to 75%. Any occupancy rate between 76% and 79% results in a loss based on the cost model.

20. **Correct Answer: B.** This statement accurately reflects the equal-pay test requirements.

21. **Correct Answer: D.** Religious beliefs and practices is the most commonly challenged category protected under this law. The law prohibits employment discrimination based on race, color, religion, sex, and national origin.

22. **Correct Answer: C.** OSHA as a law provides employees a place of employment free from recognized hazards, assures safe and healthful working conditions for men and women, and ensures employers comply with occupational safety and health standards issued in the law.

23. **Correct Answer: C.** Such an activity is within the purview of the executive. By ensuring that systems are in place to disseminate research in both nursing and management, the nurse executive helps set expectations for the organization's leadership group.

24. **Correct Answer: A.** Managers are responsible for knowing the legalities and contract requirements regarding overtime. By encouraging the manager to become more familiar with the contract, the nurse executive helps the manager fulfill her or his responsibilities and adds to the manager's competency.

25. **Correct Answer: B.** The first action by the manager in the progressive discipline process is an oral warning.

26. **Correct Answer: C.** Supplying the union with information about employees is contrary to regulations governing collective bargaining activities.

27. **Correct Answer: B.** Autonomy holds that the patient's wishes are to be respected, even if her wishes are contrary to those of her family. The covenant is between patient and physician. In this case, the physician honors the patient's decision. The patient's competence to make decisions about the extent of her care is not in question.

28. **Correct Answer: B.** HIPAA requires stringent adherence to the principles of confidentiality and includes stiff penalties in the face of violation of its tenets.

29. **Correct Answer: D.** The nurse executive ensures that nursing is well represented within whatever formal framework the organization has in place to deal with ethical issues. Nursing is generally represented on the organization's multidisciplinary ethics committee. Policies and procedures are in place to guide nurses faced with ethical dilemmas in the course of their practice.

30. **Correct Answer: B.** The act stipulates that the employer remains responsible for the acts of its employees.

31. **Correct Answer: C.** Except in an emergency situation, where consent is implied, the performance of a procedure upon a patient without his or her explicit consent, or the explicit consent of his or her agent where indicated, constitutes battery on the part of the practitioner. Battery is defined as "the deliberate touching of another without authorization."

32. **Correct Answer: C.** Title VII of the Civil Rights Act of 1964 is the landmark antidiscrimination legislation of the last century.

33. **Correct Answer: A.** The responsibility for choosing or appointing members of the medical staff of a given institution rests with the governing board (board of directors) of that organization.

34. **Correct Answer: A.** The fact that the patient seeks care, or, in the case of an emergency, needs care, can be interpreted as an implied contract.

35. **Correct Answer: C.** The physician has violated the contract agreed to with the patient, regardless of whether the alternative procedure is preferable to, or more advantageous than, the procedure that the physician contracted to perform.

36. **Correct Answer: B.** The patient can reasonably expect that his broken bone will be set according to the standards of orthopedic practice. If the internal medicine physician cannot perform to this standard, then she or he should ensure that the care of the patient is transferred to someone who can practice accordingly.

37. **Correct Answer: C.** The state issues regulations pertaining to licensure of various professions.

38. **Correct Answer: B.** As legislation that affects nursing practice becomes law, nurse executives must be cognizant of the changing statutes, their impact, and the modifications that must be made in their organizations in order to comply. Nurse executives become the "translators" of legislative change for staff.

39. **Correct Answer: D.** The practice act establishes the legal boundaries for educational requirements and scope of nursing practice in any given state.

40. **Correct Answer: C.** When the state's policies are more stringent than the federal policies, the state policies predominate. The opposite is also true. More stringent legislation always "trumps" less rigorous legislation.

41. **Correct Answer: B.** Labor–management relations laws apply to nonprofits the same as they apply to for-profit organizations.

42. **Correct Answer: C.** The Americans with Disabilities Act extends beyond physical disabilities, applying to all with mental or physical impairments that limit major life activities.

43. **Correct Answer: A.** Creating new organizational visions, building cultures, and contributing to measurable results are outcomes of appreciative inquiry. The four D's of appreciative inquiry are discover, dream, design, and deliver.

44. **Correct Answer: C.** The nurse executive is responsible for recognizing and employing every available advantage to ensure an organization's success. Recognizing and utilizing the full potential of all individuals in an organization is a leadership responsibility.

45. **Correct Answer: A.** Communication skills are paramount to successful negotiations, beginning with active listening and attention to nonverbal skills.

46. **Correct Answer: B.** Managing resources effectively in a crisis environment is important to maintain operations.

47. **Correct Answer: B.** The business plan is often the sales document for the proposed project or program, answering important questions and analyzing data related to the resources necessary to implement the project or program.

48. **Correct Answer: D.** Participation in decision-making is one of the three hallmarks of organizational transparency, leading to respect and sharing of information between management and staff and to the development of trust.

49. **Correct Answer: B.** The Fair Labor Standards Act set standards for minimum wage and child labor, and requires that compensation be paid in cash or by check.

50. **Correct Answer: A.** Explanatory notes for the rating provide a well-rounded explanation to the employee of the numerical rating when citing example(s).

INDEX

INDEX

A

B

C

D

E

F

G

H

I

J

K

L

M

N

O

P

Q

R

S

T

U

V

W

Y

Z

ABOUT THE AUTHORS

Al Rundio, PhD, DNP, RN, APRN, ANP, ACNP, ACNS, CARN-AP, NEA-BC, DPNAP, is the Associate Dean for Post-Licensure Nursing Programs & CNE at Drexel University, College of Nursing & Health Professions, in Philadelphia. Dr. Rundio also practices part-time in a residential addictions treatment center in southern New Jersey. Dr. Rundio consults on various administrative topics and is an educational consultant to the American Nurses Credentialing Center. Dr. Rundio began his management career at the age of 26. He is the former Vice President of Nursing/CNO at Shore Medical Center, Somers Point, New Jersey.

Dr. Rundio resides with his family and their two Papillions, Logan and Luke, in Egg Harbor Township, New Jersey.

Virginia "Ginny" Wilson, PhD(c), MSN, RN, NEA-BC, NE-BC, has been in practice for 39 years as an RN, with experience at multiple levels of nursing administration in healthcare organizations and leadership roles, including educator, consultant, and care provider, with a focus in emergency nursing. She is an experienced national speaker for nursing leadership programs and a featured speaker for ANCC for the past 8 years. She has been published in peer-reviewed journals and texts and has developed and been faculty for continuing education modules in nursing leadership in multiple presentation venues. Her research interests include leadership development and succession planning in healthcare organizations.

Ginny has held faculty positions at the assistant professor level in various universities and colleges in New Jersey and Pennsylvania. She teaches across multiple curriculum levels specializing in leadership development topics, legal issues in health care, healthcare policy, and the business of health care.

Ginny is currently completing a doctoral program in organization and management with a specialization in leadership. She began her career in health care as a Diploma Nurse, obtained her bachelor's degree from the University of Hawaii, and her master's degree from Widener University in Chester, PA, in Nursing Administration. She is nationally certified as a Nurse Executive, at both an operational and advanced levels.

Ginny is married, lives in southern New Jersey, and enjoys reading and traveling as her balanced self-renewal activities.

42604440R10125

Made in the USA
Lexington, KY
28 June 2015